PATIENT-CENTRIC CLINICAL TRIALS

The Role of Patient Engagement

Dr Essam Abdelhakim

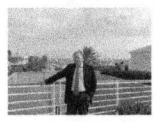

Copyright © 2024 Dr Essam Abdelhakim

All rights reserved

The characters and events portrayed in this book are fictitious. Any similarity to real persons, living or dead, is coincidental and not intended by the author.

No part of this book may be reproduced, or stored in a retrieval system, or transmitted in any form or by any means, electronic, mechanical, photocopying, recording, or otherwise, without express written permission of the publisher.

Cover design by: Art Painter
Library of Congress Control Number: 2018675309
Printed in the United States of America

CONTENTS

Title Page
Copyright
Introduction — 1
Chapter 1: Understanding the Patient Perspective — 4
Chapter 2: Patient Engagement Techniques — 11
Chapter 3: Designing Patient-Friendly Protocols — 31
Chapter 4: Implementing Decentralized and Hybrid Trial Models — 47
Chapter 5: Utilizing Patient-Reported Outcomes (PROs) — 64
Chapter 6: Enhancing Patient Support and Retention — 76
Chapter 7: Measuring and Improving Patient Experience — 89
Chapter 8: Ethical Considerations in Patient-Centric Trials — 98
Chapter 9: The Future of Patient-Centric Clinical Trials — 112
Conclusion — 124
About The Author — 129

INTRODUCTION

Definition of Patient-Centricity

Patient-centricity refers to a model of healthcare and clinical research that places patients at the center of decision-making processes, recognizing them as active partners rather than passive participants.

In the context of clinical trials, patient-centricity involves integrating patients' perspectives, preferences, and experiences into all stages of research, from study design to execution and dissemination of results. It emphasizes collaboration with patients to ensure that trials are more relevant, accessible, and aligned with their needs and concerns.

Patient-centric approaches prioritize transparency, patient empowerment, and meaningful engagement, fostering a more inclusive and collaborative environment. This model seeks to improve patient satisfaction, adherence to treatments, and ultimately, the quality of outcomes.

Historical Context and Evolution of Clinical Trials

The evolution of clinical trials has undergone significant changes over the past century. Initially, clinical trials were highly regulated, investigator-driven processes that often viewed patients as subjects rather than partners. *Historically*, research focused on scientific advancement with little regard for the patient experience, leading to rigid protocols and limited patient input in the design and execution phases.

By the late 20th century, the introduction of Good Clinical Practice (GCP) guidelines, the establishment of regulatory bodies like the

U.S. Food and Drug Administration (FDA), and the development of institutional review boards (IRBs) marked a shift towards more ethical and regulated clinical research. However, despite these advancements, patient perspectives remained underrepresented, and trials were often designed in a top-down manner without considering the lived experiences of those who would ultimately participate in or benefit from the research.

The rise of patient advocacy movements in the late 20th and early 21st centuries, particularly in areas such as oncology, HIV/AIDS, and rare diseases, brought new attention to the importance of patient voices in research. These movements paved the way for reforms that began to emphasize patient empowerment, shared decision-making, and improved communication between researchers and trial participants.

Importance of Patient-Centric Approaches in Modern Clinical Research

In today's healthcare landscape, the shift towards patient-centricity is seen as a crucial advancement in clinical research, driven by several factors:

1. **Improved Patient Recruitment and Retention:** One of the most significant challenges in clinical research is patient recruitment and retention. Patient-centric approaches improve these rates by making trials more appealing and accessible, addressing patient concerns, and reducing barriers to participation. When trials are designed with patient input, they are more likely to meet the needs of diverse populations, leading to broader enrollment and better retention.

2. **Enhanced Relevance and Applicability of Research:**

Incorporating patient perspectives helps ensure that the outcomes being measured are meaningful to patients' everyday lives. By focusing on endpoints that matter to patients—such as quality of life, symptom management, and functional outcomes—research becomes more relevant and applicable in real-world settings.

3. **Increased Patient Adherence and Engagement:** Patient-centric trials that prioritize patient education, convenience, and comfort often see higher levels of adherence to trial protocols. Engaged patients are more likely to follow study procedures, take medications as prescribed, and participate fully in the trial, leading to more reliable data and better overall outcomes.

4. **Ethical and Social Responsibility:** There is a growing recognition that clinical research has an ethical obligation to respect and include the voices of patients, particularly those from underserved or marginalized populations. Patient-centric trials promote equity in research, ensuring that the benefits of scientific advancements are shared across all patient groups.

5. **Regulatory and Industry Support:** Regulatory bodies and pharmaceutical companies have increasingly recognized the value of patient-centric approaches. Organizations such as the FDA and European Medicines Agency (EMA) have incorporated patient input into regulatory frameworks, encouraging sponsors to engage with patients early in the trial design process. Likewise, pharmaceutical companies have begun adopting patient engagement strategies to improve the success of their trials and to better align their products with patient needs.

CHAPTER 1: UNDERSTANDING THE PATIENT PERSPECTIVE

Understanding the patient perspective is fundamental to creating a truly patient-centric approach in clinical trials. Patients are no longer passive subjects in research; they are individuals with unique needs, concerns, and preferences that must be acknowledged to optimize their participation and improve the overall success of clinical trials.

1. Patient Needs and Expectations in Clinical Trials

Patients entering clinical trials often have a complex set of needs and expectations, influenced by their health conditions, personal values, and past experiences with healthcare. Recognizing and addressing these needs is crucial for improving patient engagement and adherence throughout the trial process.

1. **Access to Information and Education:** One of the most fundamental needs patients have in clinical trials is access to clear, transparent, and comprehensive information. Before enrolling in a trial, patients want to understand the purpose, risks, and potential benefits of participation. Many patients also seek detailed information about the trial's methodology, such as the types of treatments being tested, the duration of the trial, and what their role will entail.

Unfortunately, trial information is often presented in technical jargon, which can be confusing or intimidating. This disconnect can deter potential participants or lead to misunderstandings about the trial. Patients expect trial sponsors and investigators to communicate in a way that is easy to understand and that empowers them to make informed decisions about their participation.

2. **Safety and Trust:** Patient safety is a primary concern for anyone considering participation in a clinical trial. Given the experimental nature of trials, patients may be apprehensive about potential risks or side effects. They need assurance that their well-being will be closely monitored, and that safeguards are in place to protect them. Trust is a key factor in addressing this need—patients are more likely to participate in a trial if they feel confident in the integrity and expertise of the research team.

Building trust also involves being transparent about the uncertainties of the trial and offering patients the opportunity to ask questions, voice concerns, and make informed choices about their involvement.

3. **Convenience and Practicality:** Many patients are concerned about the practical aspects of trial participation, such as the time commitment, travel requirements, and the impact on their daily lives. Trials that require frequent hospital visits, long distances of travel, or complex procedures can be burdensome, particularly for patients with limited mobility or chronic conditions.

Patients expect trials to be designed with convenience in mind, minimizing disruption to their lives. This could include offering flexible appointment times, providing local trial sites, or using technologies like telemedicine to reduce the need for in-person visits. Reducing the logistical burden on patients is a key factor in promoting participation and retention.

4. **Respect and Dignity:** Patients expect to be treated with respect and dignity throughout their

participation in a clinical trial. This includes acknowledging their role as partners in the research process, respecting their privacy and confidentiality, and ensuring they have a voice in key decisions about their care.

Trials that are overly rigid or fail to accommodate patient preferences risk alienating participants. Instead, patients want to feel valued and respected as individuals, with their preferences considered in trial design, execution, and follow-up.

5. **Outcome Relevance:** Another significant patient expectation is that the outcomes being studied in a clinical trial should be relevant to their health and well-being. Patients want to see research that prioritizes issues that matter to them—improvements in quality of life, symptom relief, and functional outcomes that have a direct impact on their daily lives.

In some trials, endpoints may be more focused on biomarkers or disease progression, which may not resonate as strongly with patients. By aligning study goals with patient-centered outcomes, researchers can ensure that their work has real-world relevance for the individuals they aim to help.

2. Common Barriers to Participation

Despite the growing emphasis on patient-centricity, several barriers still exist that prevent patients from participating in clinical trials.

Identifying and addressing these barriers is essential for improving access to trials and ensuring diverse and representative patient populations.

1. **Lack of Awareness:** A significant barrier to clinical trial participation is that many patients are simply

unaware of ongoing trials or do not have access to reliable information about them. Often, patients rely on their healthcare providers to inform them about trial opportunities, but many providers may not be up to date on available studies or may not actively promote trial participation.

In addition, some patients are unaware that clinical trials are an option for their specific condition, particularly in areas like rare diseases or emerging therapies. Improving awareness through better communication channels, including social media, patient advocacy groups, and healthcare networks, is key to overcoming this barrier.

2. **Mistrust in the Research Process:** Historical instances of unethical research practices, such as the Tuskegee Syphilis Study, have left lasting scars on public trust in clinical research, particularly among marginalized communities. Mistrust of the research process and concern over exploitation can discourage participation, especially among minority populations or those with limited access to healthcare.

To rebuild trust, trial sponsors must emphasize transparency, ethical conduct, and the involvement of diverse patient voices in all aspects of trial design and execution. Collaborating with patient advocacy groups and community organizations can help foster trust and promote greater inclusivity in clinical research.

3. **Eligibility Criteria and Health Disparities:** Strict eligibility criteria can also serve as a barrier to participation. Many trials have rigid inclusion and exclusion criteria, which may inadvertently exclude patients with comorbidities, advanced age, or other health disparities. This can be particularly problematic

in conditions like cancer, where many patients may have other underlying health conditions that disqualify them from participating in trials.

Expanding eligibility criteria and designing trials that are more inclusive can help ensure that clinical research is representative of the broader patient population and that results are generalizable to real-world settings.

4. **Financial and Logistical Barriers:** Clinical trial participation can be costly for patients, both in terms of time and financial resources. Even when trials offer compensation or reimbursements, patients may still face out-of-pocket costs such as transportation, lodging, or time off work. These financial burdens disproportionately affect lower-income patients, creating disparities in trial participation.

Addressing financial and logistical barriers requires a patient-centered approach that accounts for the diverse socioeconomic backgrounds of participants. This may involve offering transportation services, providing compensation for lost wages, or partnering with community organizations to support participants.

5. **Fear of the Unknown:** Many patients are hesitant to join clinical trials due to fear of the unknown—whether it's fear of experiencing adverse effects, the uncertainty of being assigned to a placebo group, or concerns about the long-term impact of the intervention. Patients may also worry about being "experimented on" or feel anxious about the lack of control they have in the research process.

Addressing these fears through education, transparent communication, and offering support systems, such as patient liaisons or trial navigators, can help alleviate anxiety and encourage participation.

3. The Impact of Patient Experience on Trial Outcomes

The patient experience plays a critical role in shaping the success and outcomes of clinical trials. When patients are engaged, informed, and satisfied with their experience, trial results are more likely to be reliable, robust, and applicable to real-world clinical practice.

Conversely, poor patient experiences can lead to significant challenges, such as high dropout rates, poor adherence to protocols, and skewed data.

1. **Retention and Adherence:** One of the most direct impacts of patient experience on trial outcomes is retention. Patients who have positive experiences, feel valued, and are treated as partners in the research process are more likely to complete the trial. High retention rates lead to more complete data sets, reducing the risk of biased or inconclusive results.

Adherence to trial protocols is another important factor. Patients who trust their trial team, understand the study's importance, and feel supported are more likely to follow the prescribed regimen. Poor adherence can skew trial outcomes and compromise the validity of the research.

2. **Data Integrity and Quality:** Patient experience also affects the quality of data collected during a trial. Patients who feel engaged and supported are more likely to provide accurate, timely information during data collection, such as reporting side effects or completing questionnaires. In contrast, patients who feel disconnected or disillusioned may provide less reliable data, missing key follow-up appointments or neglecting to report adverse effects.

3. **Diversity and Representativeness:** The experience of

patients from diverse backgrounds also influences the representativeness of clinical trials. When trials are designed with inclusivity in mind, they are more likely to attract a diverse patient population, ensuring that trial results reflect the needs of different demographic groups. This is crucial for generalizing trial findings to real-world patient populations and for ensuring that new treatments benefit all patients, not just a select few.

4. **Patient-Reported Outcomes and Quality of Life:** Finally, patient-centric trials often incorporate patient-reported outcomes (PROs), which are direct reports from patients about how they feel and function during the trial. These outcomes provide valuable insights into the impact of an intervention on patients' quality of life, offering a more holistic understanding of treatment benefits beyond clinical or laboratory endpoints.

Incorporating the patient perspective at every stage of clinical trials leads to more meaningful, relevant research, ultimately benefiting both patients and the scientific community.

CHAPTER 2: PATIENT ENGAGEMENT TECHNIQUES

Patient engagement is a cornerstone of patient-centric clinical trials. Engaged patients are more likely to enroll in trials, adhere to study protocols, and stay involved throughout the duration of the trial.

1. Building Trust and Rapport

Trust is fundamental to patient engagement in clinical trials. Without trust, patients may be reluctant to participate or may withdraw before the study is completed. Building a trusting relationship requires empathy, honesty, and a deep commitment to the patient's well-being.

1. **Establishing Trust from the Outset:** Building trust begins at the first point of contact with potential trial participants. From the recruitment phase, it is essential to convey that the patient's well-being is the top priority. Patients need to feel that the trial team has their best interests in mind, and this can be communicated by offering clear explanations of the trial's goals, risks, benefits, and protocols.

Introducing patients to key members of the research team early on—such as the principal investigator, clinical research coordinators, and patient liaisons—can help foster familiarity and humanize the research process. Personalized interactions, where patients can ask questions and voice concerns, build a sense of partnership between the patient and the research team.

2. **Maintaining Ongoing Relationships:** Trust-building doesn't stop after initial enrollment. Maintaining rapport throughout the trial is crucial for long-term patient engagement. Regular check-ins, both formal and informal, help maintain a sense of connection and assure the patient that they are not just a subject in a study but a valued contributor to the research.

Personalizing interactions, such as remembering a patient's preferences or medical history, can go a long way in making patients feel acknowledged and cared for. A simple gesture, such as sending reminder emails or offering flexible appointment scheduling, shows that the trial staff is mindful of the patient's life and commitments.

3. **Providing Emotional and Psychological Support:** Many patients experience fear, anxiety, or uncertainty when participating in clinical trials, especially if they are dealing with a serious illness or an experimental treatment. Offering emotional support, whether through formal counseling services or informal, empathetic conversations, can significantly improve the patient experience.

Patients may also benefit from peer support, such as connecting with other participants who have undergone similar experiences. By fostering an environment of shared experiences and mutual support, clinical trial teams can build a community that strengthens trust and engagement.

4. **Empowering Patients with Shared Decision-Making:** One of the most effective ways to build trust is by involving patients in shared decision-making. Instead of viewing patients as passive subjects, engaging them as active participants in their healthcare decisions can

enhance their sense of autonomy and ownership over their trial experience.

Offering patients options where possible—such as choosing between different treatment schedules or providing alternatives for follow-up care—can empower them. Shared decision-making demonstrates that the trial team values the patient's input and respects their preferences, further reinforcing trust and rapport.

2. Effective Communication Strategies

Clear and empathetic communication is one of the most important elements of successful patient engagement in clinical trials. Effective communication can reduce misunderstandings, alleviate patient anxiety, and promote a collaborative research environment.

1. **Using Plain Language:** Medical jargon and technical terms can be overwhelming for many patients, especially those with limited healthcare literacy. To improve comprehension, trial teams should use plain language when explaining the study's purpose, procedures, and potential risks. Information should be clear, concise, and free of unnecessary complexity.

For example, instead of saying "randomized controlled trial," researchers can explain it as "a study where participants are randomly assigned to different groups to test the effects of treatments." Simple metaphors or analogies may also help patients grasp complex concepts, such as likening the clinical trial process to a scientific experiment where different treatments are being compared.

2. **Active Listening:** Effective communication is not just about delivering information but also about actively listening to patients. Active listening involves giving

patients the time and space to express their thoughts, concerns, and questions without feeling rushed or dismissed.

Trial staff should take care to demonstrate that they are fully engaged in the conversation by maintaining eye contact, nodding, and providing verbal feedback. Reflective listening, where the listener repeats or summarizes what the patient has said to confirm understanding, can also reinforce that the patient's concerns are being heard.

3. **Tailoring Communication to Individual Needs:** Not all patients communicate in the same way, and some may require special accommodations. For example, patients with hearing impairments, limited literacy, or non-English speakers may need modified communication strategies. Providing written materials in multiple languages, offering translation services, or using visual aids can help ensure that all patients have access to the information they need to make informed decisions.

Additionally, some patients may prefer digital communication tools, such as email, SMS, or telemedicine, while others may feel more comfortable with in-person meetings. Being flexible and adapting communication methods to meet individual needs can significantly enhance patient satisfaction.

4. **Delivering Bad News with Compassion:** In some trials, patients may receive disappointing or distressing news, such as learning that they are not responding to the treatment or that their condition is worsening. How this information is communicated is critical to maintaining trust and engagement.

When delivering bad news, it's important to be honest

but also compassionate. Giving patients time to process the information and offering emotional support, such as counseling or guidance on next steps, can help them feel less isolated and more supported during difficult moments.

5. **Providing Regular Updates:** Keeping patients informed throughout the trial process is vital to maintaining their engagement. Regular updates on the progress of the trial, any changes to the study protocol, or the availability of new information can help patients feel more involved and reassured.

In longer trials, it can be helpful to provide periodic updates even when there is no new significant information, as this reassures patients that the trial is moving forward and that their contributions are valued.

3. Cultural Competence in Patient Interactions

Cultural competence refers to the ability to interact effectively with individuals from diverse cultural backgrounds. In clinical trials, cultural competence is critical for creating an inclusive and welcoming environment for all participants, particularly those from underrepresented populations.

1. **Recognizing Cultural Differences:** Cultural differences can influence how patients perceive healthcare, clinical trials, and the medical research process. For example, some cultures may have strong preferences for traditional medicine over experimental treatments, while others may have deep-seated mistrust of medical institutions due to historical exploitation.

Trial teams must recognize these cultural differences and be prepared to address them with sensitivity. Engaging with community leaders or cultural liaisons can help trial teams better understand the specific needs and concerns of different cultural groups and ensure that recruitment efforts are respectful and effective.

2. **Providing Culturally Appropriate Materials:** Educational materials, consent forms, and trial documentation should be adapted to meet the cultural and linguistic needs of participants. This may involve translating materials into different languages or reworking them to better align with cultural values and healthcare beliefs.

For example, when recruiting participants from a community where family decision-making is the norm, it may be important to provide information that can be shared with family members or offer consultations that include both the patient and their family.

3. **Training Staff on Cultural Sensitivity:** Clinical trial staff should receive training in cultural sensitivity to better interact with patients from diverse backgrounds. This training can cover topics such as implicit bias, communication styles, and the specific cultural norms of the populations they serve.

Staff should be encouraged to ask questions and seek guidance when they are unsure about how to handle cultural differences, and they should strive to create an environment where patients feel comfortable discussing their cultural needs and preferences.

4. **Engaging Community Advocates:** Partnering with community organizations, patient advocacy groups, and local healthcare providers can help trial teams build trust within diverse communities. These advocates can serve as bridges between the trial team and the community, offering insights into cultural

values and helping to recruit and retain participants from underrepresented populations.

Engaging trusted community figures can also help address any concerns or misconceptions about clinical trials, promoting greater inclusivity and patient engagement.

4. Transparency in Trial Information

Transparency is essential for building trust and engaging patients in clinical trials. Patients need to feel that they are fully informed about every aspect of the trial, from its goals to its potential risks and benefits. Lack of transparency can lead to mistrust, confusion, and disengagement.

1. **Comprehensive Informed Consent:** The informed consent process is the foundation of transparency in clinical trials. Patients must be provided with all the necessary information to make an informed decision about their participation, including a clear explanation of the trial's purpose, procedures, risks, benefits, and their rights as participants.

Informed consent should be an ongoing process, with patients receiving updated information as the trial progresses. Trial teams must ensure that consent forms are written in plain language, and that patients fully understand the implications of their participation before they sign.

2. **Disclosure of Risks and Benefits:** Patients deserve full transparency about the potential risks and benefits of participating in a clinical trial. This includes explaining both known risks and uncertainties, as well as the likelihood of experiencing adverse effects.

Transparency also involves being realistic about the potential benefits of the trial. While patients may hope for positive outcomes, it's important to communicate that the trial is an experiment, and that the treatment may not work as expected or may only offer limited benefits.

3. **Real-Time Access to Data and Results:** Providing patients with access to their own data during the trial can enhance transparency and engagement. Many patients appreciate being able to track their progress, such as seeing how their health indicators change over time. Offering patients access to their data in real-time through patient portals or regular reports fosters a sense of ownership and involvement in the trial process.

Additionally, sharing aggregate trial results with participants, whether positive or negative, demonstrates that the trial team values the patient's contribution and is committed to transparency.

4. **Explaining Trial Outcomes:** At the conclusion of the trial, it is important to provide patients with a clear explanation of the results, both for the trial as a whole and for their individual participation. This can include discussing what was learned from the trial, whether the treatment was effective, and what the next steps are for the research.

Offering post-trial consultations, where patients can ask questions about their participation or receive guidance on future treatment options, can reinforce trust and engagement even after the trial is completed.

Empowering Patients As Partners

In the evolution towards patient-centric clinical trials, there is a growing recognition that patients should not just be passive participants in the research process but active partners.

Empowering patients as partners in clinical trials involves incorporating their perspectives, needs, and preferences into every stage of the trial—from design and planning to execution and follow-up.

This approach helps create trials that are more accessible, relevant, and patient-friendly, ultimately leading to improved recruitment, retention, and outcomes.

1. Involving Patients in Trial Design and Planning

Traditionally, clinical trials have been designed by researchers and sponsors with limited input from the patients who will ultimately participate in them. However, involving patients in the early stages of trial design offers invaluable insights that can make trials more patient-centered, addressing their needs, preferences, and concerns.

1. **Co-Creation of Trial Protocols:** Including patients in the trial design process helps ensure that protocols are developed with the patient's experience in mind. By collaborating with patients from the outset, researchers can gain a better understanding of the practical challenges that patients face—such as transportation issues, time constraints, or treatment side effects—and adapt the trial protocols to minimize these burdens.

For example, patients may suggest simplifying follow-up procedures, reducing the frequency of clinic visits, or incorporating home-based monitoring systems to make participation more convenient. Input from patients can also help determine which endpoints are most meaningful to them, such as improvements in quality of life rather than just clinical outcomes.

2. **Optimizing Recruitment and Retention:** Patient involvement in the planning phase can help address

one of the most significant challenges in clinical trials: recruitment and retention. By involving patients early on, researchers can better understand what motivates or deters them from participating, enabling the design of trials that are more attractive to potential participants.

For instance, patients may advise on the wording of recruitment materials to ensure they are clear, relatable, and free of medical jargon. They can also suggest more effective recruitment strategies, such as targeting specific patient communities or utilizing social media platforms to raise awareness about the trial.

3. **Ensuring Patient Relevance and Feasibility:** One of the main goals of patient involvement in trial design is to ensure that the study is both relevant and feasible for participants. Patients can provide insights into what matters most to them in terms of outcomes, helping to refine the study's objectives to reflect real-world needs.

Additionally, patients can highlight potential barriers to participation, such as the complexity of study procedures or the location of trial sites. By addressing these concerns during the planning phase, researchers can create trials that are more accessible and manageable for participants, leading to higher enrollment and lower dropout rates.

4. **Patient-Informed Consent Process:** The informed consent process can be significantly improved by involving patients in its design. Patients can help identify areas where the consent documents may be unclear or overwhelming, ensuring that all information is presented in a way that is easily understandable. This helps foster a more transparent

and trusting relationship between researchers and participants, ensuring that patients feel fully informed before enrolling in the trial.

2. Patient Advisory Boards And Focus Groups

Creating formal structures for patient involvement, such as patient advisory boards and focus groups, allows for ongoing collaboration between patients and researchers. These groups provide a platform for patients to voice their opinions, share their experiences, and contribute to the continuous improvement of clinical trials.

1. **Patient Advisory Boards:** Patient advisory boards (PABs) are composed of patients who have direct experience with the condition being studied and who can provide valuable insights into the design and conduct of clinical trials. These boards serve as a bridge between researchers and the patient community, helping to ensure that the trial reflects the needs and preferences of its participants.

PABs can be involved in various aspects of the trial process, from reviewing study protocols to advising on patient recruitment strategies. They can also play a role in reviewing trial materials, such as patient information sheets, consent forms, and follow-up surveys, to ensure they are patient-friendly and accessible.

In addition to improving the trial design, PABs can help build trust within the patient community by demonstrating that the research team values patient input and is committed to addressing patient concerns.

2. **Focus Groups:** Focus groups are another valuable tool for gathering patient perspectives during the trial

design and planning phases. These small, facilitated discussions allow researchers to gather qualitative data on patients' attitudes, preferences, and concerns regarding clinical trials.

Focus groups can be used to explore specific issues, such as patients' willingness to undergo certain procedures, their expectations for trial outcomes, or their thoughts on the trial's scheduling and logistics. By gathering feedback from a diverse group of patients, researchers can identify potential barriers to participation and make adjustments to the trial design before it is launched.

3. **Engaging Diverse Patient Voices:** It is essential that both patient advisory boards and focus groups are diverse, representing a broad range of experiences, demographics, and cultural backgrounds. This ensures that the insights gathered reflect the needs of different patient populations, including those from underrepresented groups who may face unique challenges in participating in clinical trials.

Engaging patients from diverse communities also helps ensure that the trial is designed to be inclusive and equitable, with tailored recruitment and retention strategies that address the specific barriers faced by different patient groups.

4. **Benefits of Ongoing Collaboration:** Patient advisory boards and focus groups offer a long-term approach to patient engagement. Rather than limiting patient involvement to the initial design phase, these groups can provide continuous feedback throughout the trial, helping to identify and address issues as they arise.

Ongoing collaboration with patient groups helps build a sense of partnership between patients and researchers, reinforcing trust and ensuring that the trial remains responsive to patient needs throughout its duration.

3. Continuous Feedback Mechanisms

To fully empower patients as partners, clinical trial teams must implement continuous feedback mechanisms that allow patients to share their experiences and suggestions at every stage of the trial. Feedback loops create a dynamic, two-way communication process that improves patient satisfaction, enhances trial efficiency, and ensures that patient concerns are addressed in real-time.

1. **Patient Surveys and Questionnaires:** Patient-reported outcomes (PROs) are an essential component of patient-centric trials. These surveys and questionnaires are designed to capture patients' experiences, preferences, and perceptions throughout the trial, from recruitment to post-trial follow-up.

PROs can cover a wide range of topics, including patients' perceptions of the trial's procedures, their physical and emotional well-being, and any challenges they face in adhering to the study protocol. By regularly collecting and analyzing this feedback, trial teams can make data-driven adjustments to improve the patient experience, such as modifying study visits, adjusting dosing schedules, or offering additional support services.

2. **Digital Feedback Platforms:** Advances in technology have made it easier to collect real-time feedback from patients through digital platforms. Mobile apps, patient portals, and online dashboards allow patients to report their experiences and concerns in real-time, providing trial teams with immediate insights into potential issues.

These digital tools can also be used to monitor patient adherence to study protocols and track patient-reported outcomes, offering researchers a wealth of data to improve trial efficiency and patient satisfaction.

3. **Regular Check-Ins and Touchpoints:** Establishing regular check-ins with trial participants, either in person or through virtual means, allows researchers to stay connected with patients throughout the trial. These touchpoints provide an opportunity to gather informal feedback, address any emerging issues, and offer support to patients who may be struggling with trial procedures or side effects.

By maintaining consistent communication with participants, researchers can ensure that patients feel heard and valued, fostering long-term engagement and reducing the likelihood of dropout.

4. **Adapting the Trial Based on Feedback:** A key component of continuous feedback is the ability to adapt the trial in response to patient input. Whether it's simplifying a procedure, offering additional support, or providing more frequent updates, acting on patient feedback demonstrates that the trial team is committed to creating a positive and responsive trial environment.

Patients are more likely to stay engaged and motivated if they see that their feedback is being taken seriously and that changes are being made to improve their experience. Flexibility and responsiveness are crucial for maintaining patient trust and satisfaction throughout the trial.

Leveraging Technology For Engagement

Technology has revolutionized the way clinical trials are conducted, offering new and innovative methods to engage patients throughout the research process. Digital tools such as mobile apps, patient portals, social media platforms, and even gamification have opened up avenues to increase patient participation, enhance communication, and improve adherence to study protocols.

These technologies provide convenience, personalization, and real-time engagement, making trials more accessible and patient-centric.

1. Mobile Apps and Patient Portals

Mobile apps and patient portals have become powerful tools for connecting patients with trial teams and simplifying the overall trial experience. By allowing participants to access trial information, monitor their health, and communicate with researchers in real time, these technologies can greatly improve patient engagement and retention.

   1. **Convenience and Accessibility:** Mobile apps provide patients with easy access to trial-related information and resources at their fingertips. Participants can use these apps to track their progress, complete surveys or questionnaires, and receive reminders for appointments, medications, or study tasks. The convenience of being able to engage with the trial from home or on the go significantly reduces the burden on participants, making it easier for them to remain compliant and engaged.

   Similarly, patient portals offer a centralized platform where patients can view their medical data, access study materials, and communicate directly with the trial team.

Portals can provide participants with personalized study schedules, updates on their trial progress, and important documents, such as consent forms and study guides.

2. **Real-Time Data Collection:** Mobile apps equipped with sensors, wearables, or self-reporting tools allow for real-time data collection, providing researchers with continuous insights into patients' health and experiences. These apps can collect data on vital signs, physical activity, medication adherence, and patient-reported outcomes, all of which contribute to a more comprehensive understanding of the trial's impact.

Real-time data collection not only enhances the accuracy of the study but also allows for immediate adjustments if patients experience adverse events or difficulties adhering to the trial protocol. By monitoring patients in real time, researchers can quickly intervene to ensure patient safety and maintain engagement.

3. **Personalization and Customization:** Mobile apps and patient portals can be customized to meet the specific needs and preferences of individual patients. Personalized reminders, educational content, and health tips can be tailored to each participant's condition, treatment plan, and lifestyle, ensuring that the trial remains relevant and engaging.

For example, an app might provide tailored exercise recommendations for patients participating in a trial for a new arthritis medication or deliver nutrition advice to participants in a weight-loss study. This personalized approach makes the trial feel more patient-centered and helps foster a deeper connection between participants and the study objectives.

4. **Improved Communication and Support:** Mobile apps

and patient portals facilitate two-way communication between patients and the research team. Participants can ask questions, report side effects, or provide feedback through secure messaging systems, ensuring that they feel supported throughout the trial. The ability to communicate directly with healthcare professionals also builds trust and encourages patients to remain engaged.

Additionally, these platforms can be used to deliver educational content, such as videos, articles, and infographics, that help patients better understand the trial and its goals. By empowering participants with knowledge, mobile apps and portals enhance the sense of partnership and investment in the trial.

2. Social Media and Digital Communities

Social media platforms and digital communities offer unique opportunities for trial recruitment, engagement, and support. These platforms enable researchers to reach broader and more diverse populations, while also fostering a sense of community among participants.

1. **Recruitment and Awareness:** Social media platforms, such as Facebook, Twitter, LinkedIn, and Instagram, have become powerful tools for recruiting participants to clinical trials. Researchers can target specific patient populations based on demographics, health conditions, and interests, allowing for more efficient and tailored recruitment strategies.

Through social media campaigns, researchers can raise awareness about ongoing clinical trials, share information about the study's goals and benefits, and provide details on how to enroll. Engaging content such as videos, testimonials, or infographics can capture attention and encourage potential participants to learn more about the trial.

2. **Building Digital Communities:** Digital communities, whether hosted on social media platforms or through dedicated online forums, provide patients with a space to connect with others who are participating in the same trial or who share similar health conditions. These communities foster peer support, allowing participants to share experiences, ask questions, and provide encouragement throughout the trial process.

Digital communities also serve as a valuable resource for researchers, offering insights into patient concerns, motivations, and feedback. By observing these online interactions, researchers can identify potential issues with the trial design or execution and make adjustments to improve the patient experience.

3. **Enhancing Patient Retention:** Social media and online communities help keep patients engaged and motivated throughout the trial. Regular updates, educational content, and success stories can be shared to maintain interest and commitment. By feeling connected to a larger community, patients are more likely to stay involved in the study and adhere to the trial protocol.

Additionally, online platforms can be used to celebrate patient milestones, such as completing a phase of the trial, further reinforcing the patient's sense of achievement and participation.

4. **Patient Advocacy and Awareness:** Social media provides a platform for patient advocacy groups and influencers to raise awareness about specific clinical trials or conditions. These voices can play a significant

role in encouraging participation by sharing personal stories, offering advice, and promoting the benefits of clinical research.

3. Gamification in Clinical Trials

Gamification—the application of game-design elements such as points, challenges, and rewards to non-game contexts—has emerged as an innovative strategy to boost patient engagement in clinical trials. By turning trial participation into a rewarding and interactive experience, gamification helps increase motivation, adherence, and retention.

1. **Increased Motivation:** Gamification uses elements such as point systems, leaderboards, and achievements to create a sense of competition and accomplishment. Participants can earn points or badges for completing study tasks, attending appointments, or adhering to medication schedules. These rewards provide immediate positive reinforcement, encouraging patients to stay on track and remain engaged throughout the trial.

For example, a mobile app might offer participants a virtual trophy for completing their daily medication doses or provide points for attending all scheduled study visits on time. These small rewards can make trial participation more enjoyable and less burdensome.

2. **Engagement Through Challenges:** Gamified clinical trials often introduce challenges or goals that participants can work towards. These challenges can be tailored to individual patients based on their health condition, treatment plan, or lifestyle, adding an element of fun and excitement to the trial experience.

For example, participants in a weight-loss trial might be encouraged to complete weekly fitness challenges or track their steps using a wearable device. By turning health behaviors into engaging activities, gamification promotes active participation and fosters a positive relationship with the trial process.

3. **Tracking Progress and Achievements:** Gamified platforms allow participants to track their progress and monitor their achievements over time. Visual dashboards and progress bars provide a clear picture of how far they've come in the trial and what they have accomplished, boosting their sense of achievement.

By offering continuous feedback on their performance, participants feel more in control of their involvement and are motivated to complete the trial successfully. This tracking can be particularly beneficial for long-term studies, where maintaining engagement over extended periods can be challenging.

4. **Improving Retention Rates:** The interactive and rewarding nature of gamified trials can significantly improve retention rates. Participants are more likely to remain in the study if they feel engaged and enjoy the process. Gamification also helps reduce dropout rates by providing incentives for continued participation, such as unlocking new challenges or receiving tangible rewards like gift cards or vouchers.

In some cases, gamification can also be used to encourage friendly competition between participants, further motivating them to stay involved and meet their study goals.

CHAPTER 3: DESIGNING PATIENT-FRIENDLY PROTOCOLS

A major barrier to participation in clinical trials is the complexity of trial protocols. Lengthy visits, frequent appointments, and invasive procedures can deter patients from enrolling or completing a trial. To create more patient-centric studies, it is essential to design protocols that prioritize participant convenience and comfort. Simplifying trial procedures, reducing the burden on patients, and offering flexible options can significantly improve patient recruitment, retention, and overall experience.

1. Simplifying Trial Procedures

One of the most effective ways to make clinical trials more patient-centric is by simplifying trial procedures. Complex protocols often involve multiple steps, extensive documentation, and intricate testing schedules, which can overwhelm patients. By streamlining these processes, researchers can make participation more manageable for patients, increasing the likelihood of adherence and reducing the dropout rate.

1. **Clear and Concise Documentation:** Patients are often required to review long and technical consent forms and trial documentation, which can be confusing or intimidating. To enhance patient understanding and trust, trial materials should be written in clear, non-technical language that patients can easily comprehend. Visual aids, such as infographics and diagrams, can also help explain key points and improve overall clarity.

Simplifying consent forms not only improves patient comprehension but also empowers participants to make informed decisions about their involvement in the trial. Shorter, clearer forms can help reduce the perception of risk and increase patient confidence in the trial process.

2. **Streamlining Data Collection:** Collecting data from patients is a critical aspect of clinical trials, but excessive or redundant data collection can create unnecessary burdens. By identifying key metrics and focusing on the most relevant data points, researchers can streamline data collection processes, minimizing the time and effort required from participants.

For example, researchers can limit the frequency of surveys or questionnaires to the most critical points in the study or consolidate multiple assessments into a single, comprehensive evaluation. Using digital tools such as mobile apps or wearables for real-time data collection can also reduce the need for repeated in-person visits.

3. **Simplified Trial Design:** Simplifying the trial design itself can also improve patient participation. Multi-arm trials, complex randomization procedures, or intricate dosing regimens can confuse patients and increase the risk of non-compliance. Whenever possible, trial designs should be straightforward, with clear instructions for patients on how to follow the protocol.

Researchers should also consider simplifying the criteria for eligibility and enrollment. Complicated inclusion and exclusion criteria can make it difficult for patients to understand whether they qualify for the study. A more streamlined enrollment process ensures that patients feel confident and supported from the outset.

2. Reducing Visit Frequency and Duration

Frequent visits to trial sites are a common reason for patient dropout, especially for those who live far from the research center, have demanding schedules, or face mobility challenges. Reducing the number of visits and the amount of time patients spend at each appointment can make trials more convenient and patient-friendly.

1. **Reducing the Number of In-Person Visits:** One way to reduce the burden of frequent visits is to minimize the need for in-person appointments by utilizing remote or virtual visits when appropriate. Telemedicine consultations, video check-ins, and the use of home-based monitoring devices allow patients to participate in a trial without the need to travel to a trial site for every check-up.

For example, remote visits can be scheduled for routine assessments such as symptom reporting or follow-up discussions, while in-person visits can be reserved for more critical evaluations, such as laboratory tests or imaging studies. This hybrid model of care allows for flexibility and reduces the strain on patients.

2. **Streamlining the Duration of Visits:** In addition to reducing the frequency of visits, researchers can also work to shorten the duration of each appointment. Long, multi-hour visits can be exhausting for patients and may interfere with their daily activities or responsibilities. By breaking up assessments into smaller tasks or focusing only on the most critical procedures during each visit, trial teams can reduce the time commitment required from participants.

Pre-visit preparations, such as completing questionnaires or providing home-based health data in advance, can also help reduce the time spent at the site. Providing patients with clear instructions ahead of time ensures that visits run smoothly and efficiently.

3. **Decentralized and At-Home Trial Options:** The rise of decentralized trials, where assessments and data collection occur at the patient's home or local healthcare facilities, further reduces the need for patients to travel long distances to centralized trial sites. In decentralized models, nurses or study coordinators can visit patients at home for specific tests or procedures, or patients may use mail-in kits for laboratory samples.

Decentralized trials increase accessibility, particularly for patients who have mobility limitations, live in rural areas, or have demanding personal or work schedules. By reducing the physical and logistical barriers to participation, decentralized models can significantly enhance patient engagement.

3. Minimizing Invasive Procedures

Invasive procedures, such as biopsies, blood draws, or injections, are often necessary for collecting critical trial data, but they can also be a significant source of discomfort, anxiety, and reluctance for participants. To make clinical trials more patient-centric, it is important to minimize the use of invasive procedures whenever possible and seek alternative methods for data collection.

1. **Reducing the Frequency of Invasive Procedures:** In cases where invasive procedures are necessary, trial teams should work to minimize their frequency. For example, rather than requiring weekly blood draws, researchers may be able to reduce the frequency to monthly or biweekly assessments if it doesn't compromise data integrity. Using existing health records or previously collected samples may also help

limit the need for additional invasive procedures.

Reducing the number of invasive interventions not only improves patient comfort but also helps alleviate fears associated with trial participation, such as concerns about pain or medical complications.

2. **Non-Invasive Alternatives:** Advancements in medical technology have enabled the development of non-invasive or minimally invasive alternatives for data collection. For example, wearable devices, such as smartwatches or fitness trackers, can monitor vital signs, physical activity, and sleep patterns without requiring the patient to undergo regular invasive testing.

Similarly, non-invasive imaging techniques, such as ultrasound or MRI, can provide detailed information on a patient's condition without the need for biopsies or other invasive diagnostic tests. Incorporating these alternatives into trial protocols allows patients to participate in studies with less physical discomfort.

3. **Patient Education and Support:** For procedures that cannot be avoided, providing clear information and support to patients can reduce anxiety and increase their willingness to participate. Educating patients about the purpose of each procedure, its potential risks and benefits, and the steps taken to ensure their safety helps build trust and reduces the psychological burden associated with invasive interventions.

Offering options such as local anesthesia, distraction techniques, or psychological support during invasive procedures can further enhance the patient experience.

4. Flexible Scheduling Options

Flexibility in scheduling is another key aspect of designing patient-friendly protocols. Many patients have busy lives, including work, family, and other commitments that may interfere with their ability to adhere to rigid trial schedules. Offering flexible scheduling options allows patients to participate in clinical trials without feeling overwhelmed or burdened by time constraints.

1. **Evening and Weekend Appointments:** Offering trial visits outside of traditional business hours, such as evening or weekend appointments, can significantly improve accessibility for working professionals, students, or caregivers. This flexibility allows patients to fit trial participation around their personal schedules without needing to take time off work or arrange childcare.

2. **Patient-Driven Scheduling:** Allowing patients to choose their preferred appointment times gives them a greater sense of control over the trial process. For example, patients may be given the option to select specific dates and times for each visit or reschedule appointments if conflicts arise.

Patient-driven scheduling systems, especially those integrated with mobile apps or patient portals, offer convenience and autonomy, which can improve compliance and reduce the risk of missed appointments.

3. **Home-Based and Virtual Visits:** As discussed earlier, incorporating home-based or virtual visits into the trial design offers another level of flexibility for patients. By enabling remote check-ins or sending study staff to the patient's home for certain assessments, trial teams can accommodate participants' individual needs and reduce the logistical challenges of participation.

Enhancing Protocol Readability

One of the key challenges in clinical trials is ensuring that patients fully understand the trial protocols and associated documents. Often, clinical trial materials such as consent forms, instructions, and patient guides are written in highly technical or legalistic language that can overwhelm and confuse participants. Enhancing the readability of these materials is essential to fostering trust, improving patient comprehension, and ensuring informed decision-making.

Protocols that are easy to read and understand help patients feel more comfortable and confident in participating, leading to better recruitment, engagement, and retention.

1. Using Plain Language in Patient-Facing Documents

Clinical trial documents are often filled with complex medical terminology, scientific jargon, and technical descriptions that can be difficult for non-medical participants to understand. To improve readability and patient comprehension, trial teams should prioritize the use of plain language in all patient-facing materials.

1. **Clear and Simple Vocabulary:** The goal of plain language is to convey information clearly and concisely, using words and phrases that are easy for the average reader to understand. This involves replacing complex medical terms with simpler, more commonly used alternatives. For example, instead of "adverse events," the term "side effects" may be used, or instead of "placebo," the phrase "inactive treatment" might be more easily understood. When technical terms are necessary, they should be clearly defined using straightforward language.

   Avoiding overly long sentences and limiting the use of

acronyms or abbreviations can also enhance clarity. Sentences should be short, active, and direct, with one main idea per sentence to ensure easy comprehension.

2. **Accessible Formatting:** The way information is presented on the page also impacts readability. Documents should be well-organized, with headings and subheadings that clearly indicate different sections or topics. Bullet points or numbered lists can be used to break up large blocks of text and make key information easier to digest.

A readable font size (at least 12-point), sufficient line spacing, and ample margins also contribute to making documents more accessible. Bold text or colored highlights can be used to emphasize critical points, such as trial participation requirements, safety information, or consent details.

3. **Clear Objectives and Instructions:** Patients need to understand not only the purpose of the trial but also their specific role in it. Documents should explicitly state the objectives of the study in plain terms, explaining what the trial is designed to achieve and how their participation contributes to that goal.

Instructions for patients—whether related to medication regimens, data collection, or visit schedules—should be written in a step-by-step manner. Each instruction should be simple and specific, avoiding any ambiguities that could cause confusion.

2. Visual Aids and Infographics

Visual aids such as charts, diagrams, and infographics are valuable tools for enhancing understanding, particularly for patients who struggle with reading or processing large amounts of text. They can clarify complex concepts, summarize key points, and make information more memorable.

1. **Simplifying Complex Concepts:** Many aspects of clinical trials, such as randomization, the use of placebos, or multi-arm study designs, can be difficult for patients to grasp through text alone. Diagrams or flowcharts can help visualize these concepts, showing how patients are assigned to different treatment groups, what the different trial phases entail, or how a particular intervention is administered.

For example, a flowchart could show the steps of trial participation—from screening and randomization to treatment and follow-up visits—providing a clear and intuitive overview of what to expect. Similarly, a graph could illustrate how the study drug is expected to affect patients over time compared to a placebo.

2. **Infographics for Key Takeaways:** Infographics combine visuals and concise text to deliver key information in an easily digestible format. For clinical trials, infographics can be used to summarize trial objectives, potential benefits and risks, patient responsibilities, and safety measures. Infographics work particularly well for conveying critical information such as dosage instructions, side effect monitoring, or emergency contact procedures.

A well-designed infographic can also alleviate concerns or fears by showing what will happen during certain procedures (e.g., blood draws, MRIs) in a clear, non-threatening way.

3. **Timelines and Visit Schedules:** Timelines are another helpful visual tool, particularly when patients are required to attend multiple visits or undergo certain procedures at specific times. A timeline graphic can

visually display important milestones in the trial, such as when treatment phases begin and end, when lab tests are needed, or when patients can expect follow-up assessments.

Visualizing the schedule in this way helps patients better understand what to expect and how to plan their time accordingly, reducing the risk of missed appointments or non-compliance.

3. Multilingual Resources

In clinical trials, it is essential to ensure that all patients, regardless of language proficiency, can fully understand and engage with the trial materials. Providing multilingual resources tailored to the linguistic and cultural needs of diverse populations can help increase participation and improve the overall patient experience.

1. **Translations of Trial Materials:** Clinical trial documents, including consent forms, instructions, and informational brochures, should be translated into the primary languages spoken by the target patient population. This ensures that non-English-speaking patients can fully understand the purpose of the trial, the potential risks and benefits, and their rights and responsibilities as participants.

It is important to use professional, culturally sensitive translation services to ensure accuracy and clarity. Machine translations or poorly translated documents can lead to misunderstandings or misinterpretations, putting patient safety at risk and potentially compromising the trial's integrity.

2. **Culturally Adapted Materials:** Beyond simple translation, patient-facing materials should be culturally adapted to reflect the values, beliefs, and practices of the populations being recruited. Certain

medical concepts or procedures may carry different connotations or levels of acceptability across cultures, so it's important to present information in a way that resonates with patients' backgrounds.

Cultural adaptation also extends to the design and tone of materials. For instance, illustrations or photographs included in trial documents should reflect the diversity of the patient population, ensuring that patients see themselves represented in the materials.

3. **Bilingual Trial Staff:** In addition to multilingual written materials, having bilingual staff available at trial sites can enhance communication and patient support. Bilingual research coordinators or interpreters can provide real-time assistance, helping patients navigate trial procedures, answer questions, or clarify any doubts that arise during participation.

Verbal communication is often critical for ensuring that patients feel comfortable and supported, particularly when dealing with complex or sensitive topics such as informed consent or medical procedures.

Incorporating Patient Input

Incorporating patient input into clinical trials is a cornerstone of patient-centric research. By actively involving patients in the design and evaluation of trials, researchers can ensure that studies are more aligned with patient priorities, resulting in better engagement, improved recruitment, and more meaningful outcomes. Key strategies for incorporating patient input include the use of patient-reported endpoints, quality of life assessments, and balancing scientific rigor with patient preferences.

1. Patient-Reported Endpoints (PREs)

Patient-reported endpoints (PREs) are outcomes reported directly by patients about their health status, symptoms, and the impact of treatment, without interpretation by clinicians or researchers. These endpoints are critical in assessing how patients themselves experience the benefits or side effects of a therapy, providing a more comprehensive understanding of the treatment's real-world impact.

1. **Capturing Patient-Centered Data:** PREs offer insights into how treatments affect patients' day-to-day lives, addressing aspects such as symptom relief, physical functioning, emotional well-being, and treatment burden. These outcomes are often more reflective of patient priorities compared to traditional clinical endpoints like lab values or imaging results. For instance, while a clinician may focus on tumor size reduction in a cancer trial, a patient may prioritize their ability to manage fatigue or maintain mobility.

By incorporating PREs, researchers can ensure that clinical trials measure not only objective medical outcomes but also the subjective experiences that matter most to patients.

2. **Tools for Collecting PREs:** PREs are typically collected through validated questionnaires and surveys that patients complete at various points throughout the trial. These tools might ask patients to rate their pain levels, describe how their condition affects daily activities, or report on their mental health.

Common tools for measuring PREs include the Patient-Reported Outcomes Measurement Information System (PROMIS), the EuroQol 5-Dimension (EQ-5D) scale, and disease-specific instruments like the Asthma Quality of Life Questionnaire (AQLQ).

These tools allow patients to provide detailed feedback on the specific challenges they face, which can be used to tailor treatments or adjust trial protocols to better meet patient needs.

3. **Impact on Regulatory Approvals:** The growing recognition of the importance of PREs is reflected in regulatory guidelines, with agencies like the U.S. Food and Drug Administration (FDA) and the European Medicines Agency (EMA) encouraging their inclusion in clinical trials. PREs can help demonstrate a treatment's value from a patient's perspective, influencing regulatory approvals, reimbursement decisions, and even clinical practice guidelines.

2. Quality of Life Assessments

Quality of life (QoL) assessments are another vital component of patient-centric clinical trials. These assessments measure the overall well-being of patients, taking into account not only physical health but also emotional, social, and psychological factors.

Trials that prioritize QoL assessments aim to ensure that treatments not only prolong life but also improve the quality of that life.

1. **Holistic Evaluation of Treatment Impact:** Quality of life assessments allow researchers to understand how treatments affect patients beyond traditional clinical outcomes. For example, a cancer therapy may extend survival, but if it causes debilitating side effects like nausea or chronic fatigue, the patient's quality of life may be significantly diminished. QoL assessments provide a broader picture of the treatment's impact on the patient's physical and emotional well-being, social interactions, and daily functioning.

2. **Standardized QoL Instruments:** Commonly used QoL assessment tools include the SF-36 Health Survey, the European Organization for Research and Treatment of Cancer Quality of Life Questionnaire (EORTC QLQ-C30), and the Functional Assessment of Cancer Therapy (FACT) scales. These tools help evaluate factors such as pain levels, energy, social relationships, and mental health, offering a multidimensional view of patient well-being.

QoL assessments are particularly important in trials for chronic conditions or terminal illnesses, where the goal may not only be to cure or manage the disease but also to optimize the patient's remaining quality of life.

3. **Improving Patient Engagement:** Including QoL assessments can improve patient engagement by making patients feel that their overall well-being is a priority in the trial. Knowing that their comfort and happiness are being measured and valued can foster greater trust and participation. Patients may be more likely to stay enrolled in trials if they believe that their quality of life is being actively monitored and addressed.

3. Balancing Scientific Rigor with Patient Preferences

While patient input is invaluable, it must be balanced with the need for scientific rigor in clinical trials. Incorporating patient preferences in trial design can sometimes pose challenges, particularly when patients' desires for convenience or comfort conflict with the stringent requirements needed to generate reliable data. Striking the right balance ensures that trials remain scientifically valid while also being patient-friendly.

1. **Flexible Protocol Design:** One approach to balancing rigor with patient preferences is incorporating flexibility into trial protocols. This could include

offering patients different options for how they participate, such as attending in-person visits versus remote check-ins via telemedicine. Similarly, allowing patients to choose time slots for appointments or providing transportation assistance can make trials more accessible without compromising the scientific validity of the study.

2. **Patient-Centered Outcomes with Traditional Endpoints:** Researchers can design studies that measure both traditional clinical endpoints (such as disease progression, biomarkers, or survival) and patient-centered outcomes (such as symptom burden or QoL). This dual approach ensures that the trial captures both scientifically rigorous data and patient-relevant insights, leading to more holistic conclusions about the efficacy and safety of a treatment.

For example, in a trial for a new diabetes medication, clinical endpoints might include HbA1c levels and fasting glucose, while patient-reported outcomes could focus on energy levels, ease of managing symptoms, and overall quality of life.

3. **Continuous Feedback Loops:** To maintain a balance between rigor and patient preferences, clinical trials can incorporate continuous feedback mechanisms where patients regularly provide input on their experiences. This feedback can be used to make real-time adjustments to the protocol—such as revising visit schedules, addressing unexpected side effects, or altering data collection methods—without compromising the integrity of the trial. These adaptive trial designs allow flexibility while still generating high-quality, reliable data.

CHAPTER 4: IMPLEMENTING DECENTRALIZED AND HYBRID TRIAL MODELS

The landscape of clinical trials is evolving rapidly, with decentralized clinical trials (DCTs) and hybrid trial models offering innovative ways to conduct research. These approaches aim to reduce the burden on patients and increase accessibility, while maintaining the integrity of the scientific process.

Overview of Decentralized Clinical Trials (DCTs)

Decentralized clinical trials (DCTs) refer to clinical studies in which certain or all aspects of the trial are conducted remotely, with the use of digital tools and technologies to collect data, monitor patients, and ensure compliance. Unlike traditional site-based trials, DCTs can reduce or eliminate the need for patients to visit clinical sites by leveraging telemedicine, wearable devices, mobile apps, and home health services.

1. **Key Characteristics of DCTs:**
    - **Remote Data Collection:** Participants can provide data from their homes using smartphones, wearable devices, or other sensors. Data such as heart rate, glucose levels, physical activity, and medication adherence can be captured in real-time, offering continuous insights.
    - **Telemedicine and Virtual Visits:** Rather than requiring in-person visits to clinical trial sites, DCTs often utilize video consultations, phone calls, and

online communication tools for patient assessments and follow-up visits.
- **Home-Based or Localized Services:** In some decentralized models, healthcare professionals visit the patient's home to perform clinical assessments, collect samples (such as blood or saliva), or administer treatments, reducing the need for travel to centralized trial sites.
- **Mobile and E-consent:** Participants can enroll in trials through electronic consent (e-consent) systems, which provide detailed information about the trial and allow patients to consent digitally. This process simplifies recruitment and improves the participant's understanding of the study.

2. **Hybrid Models:** Hybrid clinical trials are a blend of traditional and decentralized elements. In hybrid models, certain trial activities may be conducted remotely, such as patient monitoring or data collection, while others, such as complex procedures or diagnostic tests, require in-person visits. Hybrid models offer flexibility by combining the best of both worlds—remote convenience and hands-on care when necessary.

Benefits and Challenges of DCTs

Decentralized clinical trials offer numerous advantages for both patients and researchers, but they also introduce new challenges that must be addressed to ensure their success.

Benefits of DCTs

1. **Improved Patient Access and Diversity:** One of the most significant benefits of DCTs is the ability to reach a broader and more diverse population of participants. Patients who live in rural or underserved areas, have

mobility issues, or are unable to travel long distances for frequent clinic visits can participate in trials from the comfort of their homes. This inclusivity leads to more representative patient populations, which can improve the generalizability of trial results.

2. **Enhanced Patient Convenience and Retention:** DCTs reduce the logistical burdens associated with traditional trials, such as traveling to study sites, taking time off work, or arranging childcare. By minimizing these inconveniences, patients are more likely to enroll in and remain committed to the study, reducing dropout rates and improving trial efficiency.

3. **Real-Time Data Collection:** The use of wearable devices, mobile apps, and remote monitoring tools enables the continuous collection of real-time data. This can provide researchers with a more comprehensive understanding of how a treatment affects patients in their daily lives, beyond the limited data collected during periodic in-person visits in traditional trials.

4. **Reduced Trial Costs:** DCTs have the potential to reduce the overall cost of clinical trials by eliminating the need for large physical trial sites and staff. While there are upfront costs associated with implementing technology and logistics, decentralized models may lead to savings in areas like travel reimbursements, site monitoring, and operational expenses.

5. **Faster Recruitment and Trial Execution:** The ability to enroll participants remotely through online platforms or e-consent systems can accelerate recruitment, especially for rare diseases or geographically dispersed populations. Additionally, the flexibility and convenience of DCTs may allow trials to run more efficiently, with fewer delays due to patient scheduling conflicts or site limitations.

Challenges Of Dcts

1. **Technological Barriers:** While DCTs rely on digital tools, not all patients have access to or are comfortable using the necessary technology. Participants may lack smartphones, reliable internet access, or the skills to use wearable devices. Addressing this digital divide is crucial for ensuring equitable participation in DCTs.

2. **Data Privacy and Security Concerns:** The use of digital platforms to collect and store sensitive patient data raises concerns about privacy and security. Robust cybersecurity measures must be in place to protect participant information, comply with regulations like the General Data Protection Regulation (GDPR), and prevent data breaches.

3. **Compliance and Monitoring:** Ensuring patient compliance with study protocols in a decentralized setting can be challenging. Without direct supervision at a clinical site, researchers must rely on remote monitoring tools and self-reported data, which may not always be accurate or complete. Strategies for ensuring adherence to treatment regimens and data collection protocols must be carefully considered.

4. **Logistical and Operational Complexities:** Coordinating the logistics of home-based services, such as sample collection or drug administration, can be complex. Trials may need to partner with home healthcare providers, courier services, or local clinics, which introduces additional operational layers to manage.

5. **Investigator Oversight:** In traditional trials, investigators have direct oversight of patients during in-person visits. In decentralized models, maintaining

this level of oversight is more difficult, especially when it comes to detecting adverse events or ensuring that procedures are performed correctly in a remote setting. Alternative oversight strategies, such as telemedicine consultations or home health visits, need to be implemented.

Regulatory Considerations

As DCTs become more common, regulatory agencies are adapting to provide guidance and oversight for these innovative trial models. Sponsors and researchers must be aware of the regulatory frameworks that govern decentralized and hybrid trials, ensuring that their designs comply with local and international regulations.

1. **Regulatory Acceptance of DCTs:** Regulatory bodies like the FDA, EMA, and Health Canada have begun to embrace decentralized models, issuing guidelines that support the use of digital tools, remote monitoring, and e-consent. For example, the FDA's guidance on decentralized clinical trials encourages the use of telemedicine and remote data collection, while ensuring that patient safety and data integrity remain top priorities.

2. **Good Clinical Practice (GCP) Compliance:** Even in a decentralized environment, DCTs must adhere to the principles of Good Clinical Practice (GCP). This includes ensuring that patient safety is paramount, data is accurate and reliable, and the trial is conducted in an ethical manner. Sponsors must work closely with regulatory agencies to ensure that decentralized elements of the trial do not compromise GCP standards.

3. **Data Privacy and Security Regulations:** Protecting patient data is a critical concern in decentralized

trials. Regulatory frameworks such as the GDPR in Europe and the Health Insurance Portability and Accountability Act (HIPAA) in the U.S. impose strict requirements on the handling, storage, and sharing of personal health information. Sponsors must ensure that their digital tools and platforms are compliant with these regulations and that robust data protection measures are in place.

4. **Remote Monitoring and Safety Oversight:** In DCTs, ensuring patient safety remotely is a key regulatory consideration. Agencies require clear protocols for monitoring adverse events, providing emergency care if needed, and ensuring that participants have access to healthcare professionals throughout the trial. Sponsors must demonstrate how they will monitor patient safety and provide necessary interventions, even when patients are not visiting a central trial site.

5. **Global Regulatory Variations:** Conducting decentralized trials across multiple countries introduces additional complexity, as regulatory requirements vary from one region to another. Sponsors must navigate these differences, ensuring that they comply with each jurisdiction's rules on remote data collection, telemedicine, and patient privacy. Global harmonization of regulatory guidelines for DCTs is an ongoing effort that will help simplify the implementation of these models in the future.

Hybrid Trial Designs

Hybrid trial designs represent a flexible and innovative approach to conducting clinical research by integrating traditional and decentralized elements. This approach allows researchers to leverage the advantages of both methodologies, catering to diverse patient needs, enhancing recruitment and retention, and maintaining the scientific rigor necessary for successful trial outcomes.

Combining Traditional and Decentralized Elements

Hybrid trial designs seamlessly blend the in-person, site-based components of traditional clinical trials with the remote, patient-centric features of decentralized trials. This combination allows researchers to optimize trial protocols, improving patient experience and data collection while ensuring compliance with regulatory standards.

1. **Elements of Traditional Trials:**
    - **Site-Based Assessments:** Hybrid trials maintain essential site-based components, such as critical assessments or interventions that require direct supervision from healthcare professionals. This might include laboratory tests, complex diagnostic procedures, or administration of certain investigational products.
    - **In-Person Monitoring:** While remote monitoring is crucial in a hybrid design, certain elements necessitate in-person visits for safety evaluations, especially for complex treatments or when patients may be at risk for adverse events.
    - **Standardized Protocols:** Traditional trials often rely on well-defined protocols to

ensure uniformity across sites. Hybrid trials can retain these standardized procedures while incorporating flexibility to adapt to patient needs.

2. **Elements of Decentralized Trials:**
    - **Remote Patient Monitoring:** Hybrid designs utilize digital health technologies, such as wearable devices, mobile applications, and telehealth consultations, to collect data from patients in real-time. This allows for continuous monitoring of patient health and treatment adherence, without requiring frequent site visits.
    - **Home Health Services:** Hybrid trials can employ home healthcare professionals for procedures like sample collection, vital sign assessments, or even administering investigational products. This flexibility enables patients to participate more comfortably and conveniently.
    - **E-consent and Digital Platforms:** Patients can provide consent electronically, access study materials through patient portals, and communicate with research staff remotely, making participation more accessible and engaging.
3. **Integration of Data Collection:** Hybrid designs benefit from integrated data collection methods, combining traditional data (e.g., clinical assessments during site visits) with real-time data from remote monitoring tools. This comprehensive data approach enhances the richness of the dataset, allowing for more nuanced analysis of patient responses to treatment.

Tailoring Approaches To Specific Therapeutic Areas

The versatility of hybrid trial designs allows for tailored approaches that can address the unique challenges and requirements of specific therapeutic areas. By understanding the specific patient populations, disease characteristics, and treatment modalities involved, researchers can customize hybrid designs to optimize trial efficiency and patient engagement.

1. **Oncology Trials:**
    - **Complex Treatment Regimens:** In oncology, treatments often require close monitoring for side effects and efficacy. Hybrid trials can facilitate in-person assessments for chemotherapy infusions or radiation therapy while allowing for remote monitoring of patient symptoms and side effects through digital platforms.
    - **Longitudinal Follow-Up:** Many cancer patients undergo long-term follow-up care to assess treatment outcomes and recurrence. Hybrid models enable ongoing assessments through telehealth consultations, reducing the burden of frequent hospital visits while maintaining close patient-provider communication.

2. **Cardiovascular Trials:**
    - **Lifestyle and Behavior Monitoring:** Cardiovascular trials often focus on lifestyle factors and long-term adherence to treatment regimens. Hybrid designs can incorporate remote monitoring of physical activity, dietary habits, and medication

adherence through wearable devices and mobile health apps, while maintaining periodic site visits for crucial assessments like echocardiograms or stress tests.
- **Patient Engagement in Self-Management:** Engaging patients in their own care is critical in cardiovascular studies. Hybrid trials can employ educational components delivered via digital platforms, helping patients understand their condition and encouraging active participation in managing their health.

3. **Neurology Trials:**
   - **Symptom Tracking and Real-Time Data:** Neurological conditions such as multiple sclerosis or Parkinson's disease require careful monitoring of symptoms, which can vary significantly over time. Hybrid designs can facilitate remote symptom tracking through mobile apps, allowing for real-time reporting while scheduling in-person visits for neurological examinations and imaging studies as needed.
   - **Cognitive and Behavioral Assessments:** Hybrid trials can integrate remote cognitive assessments using digital tools, enabling patients to complete tests from home while still allowing for comprehensive evaluations during site visits.

4. **Rare Disease Trials:**
   - **Expanding Patient Access:** Rare diseases often present challenges in recruitment due to the small patient population. Hybrid designs can reach geographically dispersed

patients by providing remote assessment options, making participation feasible for individuals who might not be able to travel to a central site.

- **Tailored Patient Support:** Engaging patients with rare diseases can benefit from hybrid trials that incorporate personalized support through telehealth consultations, online resources, and local healthcare providers who can assist with patient monitoring and care.

5. **Pediatric Trials:**

    - **Family-Centric Approaches:** In pediatric trials, involving caregivers and families in the research process is crucial. Hybrid designs can offer flexibility in participation for families, allowing them to engage remotely while scheduling in-person visits for key assessments, such as physical examinations or laboratory tests.

    - **Minimizing Disruption:** Reducing the need for frequent clinic visits is particularly important for families with young children. Hybrid models enable parents to participate in trials while managing their child's routine, balancing research commitments with everyday life.

Technology Infrastructure For Remote Trials

The advent of remote clinical trials has significantly transformed the landscape of clinical research, necessitating robust technology infrastructure to facilitate effective patient engagement, data collection, and regulatory compliance. This infrastructure encompasses a variety of technological tools and systems, including telemedicine platforms, electronic consent (eConsent) systems, and remote monitoring devices and wearables. Each of these elements plays a critical role in ensuring that remote trials are efficient, patient-centric, and scientifically rigorous.

Telemedicine Platforms

Telemedicine platforms are essential for facilitating remote consultations and interactions between patients and healthcare providers. These platforms provide a virtual environment where patients can engage with clinical trial staff, receive medical advice, and participate in assessments without the need for in-person visits.

1. **Key Features of Telemedicine Platforms:**
    - **Video Conferencing:** High-quality video conferencing capabilities enable real-time consultations, allowing healthcare providers to assess patient conditions, monitor treatment responses, and provide personalized care. This is particularly beneficial for patients with mobility challenges or those living in remote areas.
    - **Secure Messaging:** Integrated messaging systems allow for asynchronous communication between patients and trial staff. Patients can ask questions, report side

effects, or request information, enhancing the ongoing dialogue throughout the trial.
- **Appointment Scheduling:** Telemedicine platforms often include scheduling tools that allow patients to book appointments conveniently. Automated reminders can help ensure patients attend virtual visits, reducing no-show rates and improving engagement.
- **Integration with Electronic Health Records (EHR):** Seamless integration with EHR systems allows trial staff to access patient medical histories, laboratory results, and medication lists, providing comprehensive insights that inform clinical decision-making during virtual visits.

2. **Benefits of Telemedicine Platforms:**
   - **Increased Access:** By eliminating the need for travel, telemedicine platforms make it easier for patients to participate in trials, especially those with rare diseases or complex medical conditions. This accessibility can lead to more diverse patient recruitment.
   - **Enhanced Patient Engagement:** Virtual interactions foster continuous engagement, empowering patients to take an active role in their healthcare. The convenience of telemedicine encourages adherence to trial protocols and follow-up assessments.
   - **Real-Time Data Collection:** Telemedicine platforms can facilitate the collection of real-time data during virtual visits, allowing researchers to track patient progress and

treatment outcomes more effectively.

Electronic Consent (Econsent) Systems

Electronic consent systems (eConsent) are a vital component of modern clinical trials, streamlining the consent process while ensuring that patients are adequately informed about their participation.

1. **Key Features of eConsent Systems:**
    - **Interactive Consent Forms:** eConsent systems often provide interactive consent forms that present information in a clear, engaging manner. These forms may include videos, infographics, and question-and-answer sections to enhance understanding.
    - **Multilingual Support:** Many eConsent systems offer multilingual options, ensuring that non-English speaking patients can comprehend the study details and make informed decisions about participation.
    - **Digital Signatures:** Patients can electronically sign consent forms, simplifying the documentation process and reducing the reliance on physical paperwork. This feature enhances data security and compliance with regulatory standards.
    - **Audit Trails:** eConsent systems maintain detailed audit trails of consent activities, including timestamps of when consent was obtained and any modifications made to the consent documents. This transparency is crucial for regulatory compliance and ethical standards.
2. **Benefits of eConsent Systems:**

- **Improved Understanding:** Interactive and visually appealing consent forms can enhance patient understanding of trial protocols, potential risks, and benefits. This clarity can lead to more informed consent and a stronger commitment to participation.
- **Efficiency and Convenience:** eConsent allows patients to review and sign consent forms from the comfort of their homes, eliminating the need for in-person visits solely for consent purposes. This convenience can reduce barriers to participation.
- **Real-Time Updates:** Researchers can quickly update consent forms to reflect changes in study protocols or new safety information. eConsent systems allow for immediate dissemination of updated information, ensuring that patients remain informed throughout the trial.

Remote Monitoring Devices And Wearables

Remote monitoring devices and wearables are integral to collecting patient data outside traditional clinical settings. These technologies enable continuous health monitoring, data collection, and timely interventions.

1. **Types of Remote Monitoring Devices:**
    - **Wearable Devices:** Wearable technologies, such as smartwatches and fitness trackers, can monitor vital signs (e.g., heart rate, blood pressure, and oxygen saturation), physical activity levels, and sleep patterns.

These devices provide valuable insights into patient health and treatment adherence.
- **Mobile Health Apps:** Mobile applications can facilitate symptom tracking, medication adherence reminders, and patient-reported outcomes (PROs). Patients can use these apps to report side effects, mood changes, or other health-related information in real time.
- **Biometric Sensors:** Devices equipped with biometric sensors can monitor specific health parameters, such as glucose levels in diabetic patients or electrocardiogram (ECG) readings in patients with cardiac conditions. These sensors provide critical data that inform treatment decisions and enhance patient safety.

2. **Benefits of Remote Monitoring Devices and Wearables:**
   - **Continuous Data Collection:** Remote monitoring allows for the collection of continuous, real-world data on patient health, providing researchers with a more comprehensive understanding of treatment effects and patient experiences.
   - **Timely Interventions:** Real-time monitoring enables healthcare providers to identify potential issues early, allowing for timely interventions that can mitigate adverse events and improve patient outcomes.
   - **Enhanced Patient Autonomy:** By empowering patients to monitor their own health, remote devices and wearables foster a sense of autonomy and engagement

in their care. Patients become active participants in their health management, contributing valuable insights to the trial process.

CHAPTER 5: UTILIZING PATIENT-REPORTED OUTCOMES (PROS)

Patient-Reported Outcomes (PROs) have emerged as a critical component of clinical research, providing invaluable insights into the patient experience and the effectiveness of interventions from the patient's perspective. By systematically capturing patient feedback on their health status, symptoms, and quality of life, researchers can enhance the relevance and applicability of their findings.

Importance Of Pros In Clinical Research

1. **Definition and Scope of PROs:** Patient-Reported Outcomes refer to any report of the status of a patient's health condition that comes directly from the patient, without interpretation by healthcare providers or anyone else. This can include a variety of metrics such as symptom severity, functional status, and overall health-related quality of life (HRQoL).

2. **Enhancing Patient-Centricity:** Incorporating PROs into clinical trials aligns with the shift towards patient-centric research. By valuing patient perspectives, researchers can better understand how diseases and treatments affect individuals' lives, ultimately leading to more relevant and meaningful outcomes.

3. **Regulatory Emphasis:** Regulatory agencies, including the FDA and EMA, increasingly recognize the importance of PROs. Guidance documents encourage

the inclusion of patient-reported data to support claims of efficacy and safety in new therapies. This regulatory focus underscores the legitimacy and necessity of PROs in the clinical research process.

4. **Informing Treatment Decisions:** PROs provide insights into the effectiveness of treatments as experienced by patients. By understanding patients' perceptions of their health and treatment outcomes, healthcare providers can make more informed decisions tailored to individual needs and preferences.

Capturing The Patient Voice

1. **Direct Insights from Patients:** PROs are invaluable in capturing the nuances of patient experiences, including the impact of symptoms on daily activities, emotional well-being, and overall quality of life. These insights are often missed when relying solely on clinical assessments conducted by healthcare professionals.

2. **Patient Engagement and Empowerment:** Involving patients in reporting their outcomes fosters a sense of ownership over their health journey. When patients contribute their perspectives, they become active participants in their care, enhancing engagement and adherence to treatment protocols.

3. **Tailored Measurements:** Developing PRO measures that are specific to the patient population and disease in question ensures that the data collected accurately reflect patient experiences. Utilizing validated PRO instruments enhances the credibility and reliability of the data, enabling researchers to draw meaningful conclusions.

4. **Feedback Loops:** Incorporating mechanisms for

continuous feedback allows researchers to make real-time adjustments to trials based on patient input. This iterative approach ensures that the study remains aligned with patient needs and experiences throughout its duration.

Complementing Traditional Clinical Endpoints

1. **Holistic Evaluation of Treatment Effects:** While traditional clinical endpoints, such as survival rates and disease progression, remain essential, they often fail to capture the full spectrum of treatment effects on patients' lives. PROs fill this gap by providing complementary data that reflects how patients perceive their health, allowing for a more holistic evaluation of treatment effectiveness.

2. **Understanding Treatment Burdens:** PROs can help identify the burdens associated with treatment, including side effects and impacts on daily functioning. This understanding is critical for assessing the trade-offs between treatment benefits and potential detriments, guiding clinicians and patients in shared decision-making.

3. **Informing Regulatory and Reimbursement Decisions:** The integration of PROs into clinical trials can strengthen the evidence base for regulatory submissions and reimbursement requests. Demonstrating that a treatment improves quality of life or reduces symptom burden can be influential in securing approvals and coverage decisions.

4. **Enhancing Study Relevance:** By incorporating PROs, researchers can ensure that study outcomes resonate with the patient population. This alignment increases the relevance of research findings, making them more likely to be adopted into clinical practice.

Designing Effective Pro Measures

Designing effective Patient-Reported Outcome (PRO) measures is critical for capturing meaningful data that reflects patients' experiences and perceptions regarding their health and treatment outcomes.

Selecting Appropriate Pro Instruments

1. **Identifying Relevant Domains:** The first step in designing PRO measures is to identify the key domains that are relevant to the specific patient population and health condition being studied. Domains may include symptoms, functional status, emotional well-being, and health-related quality of life (HRQoL). Engaging stakeholders—such as patients, healthcare providers, and researchers—can help ensure that the selected domains reflect the patient perspective.

2. **Choosing Established Instruments:** Whenever possible, researchers should opt for existing, validated PRO instruments that have demonstrated effectiveness in similar populations. Established tools come with a wealth of empirical data supporting their use, which can save time and resources in the development process. Instruments like the EQ-5D, SF-36, and PROMIS measures are commonly used across various health conditions.

3. **Tailoring Instruments for Specific Conditions:** While established instruments can provide a solid foundation, it is essential to tailor them to the specific context of the clinical trial. This may involve adding or modifying items to capture nuances related to the

particular disease, treatment, or patient demographic. Customization should be done carefully to ensure that it does not compromise the instrument's validity.

4. **Engaging Patients in Development:** Involving patients in the development and selection of PRO measures ensures that the chosen instruments accurately reflect their experiences. This collaboration can be achieved through focus groups, interviews, or surveys, allowing patients to provide input on which aspects of their health and well-being they consider most important to measure.

Ensuring Validity And Reliability

1. **Establishing Validity:** Validity refers to the extent to which a PRO measure accurately captures the construct it intends to measure. There are several types of validity to consider:
   - **Content Validity:** Ensures that the items included in the measure are relevant and representative of the construct. This can be assessed through expert review and patient input.
   - **Construct Validity:** Determines whether the PRO measure correlates with other measures as theoretically expected. For example, a PRO measure assessing pain should correlate with clinical assessments of pain severity.
   - **Criterion Validity:** Examines the relationship between the PRO measure and a gold standard or established measure, providing evidence that the new measure performs similarly.
2. **Assessing Reliability:** Reliability refers to the

consistency of a PRO measure over time and across different contexts. Key aspects of reliability include:

- **Internal Consistency:** Assesses whether the items within the PRO measure consistently measure the same construct. This can be evaluated using statistical methods such as Cronbach's alpha.
- **Test-Retest Reliability:** Measures the stability of the PRO instrument over time. Patients should yield similar scores when completing the measure on different occasions, provided that their health status has not changed.
- **Inter-Rater Reliability:** Evaluates the consistency of scores assigned by different raters or assessors when applicable, ensuring that the measure is objective and reliable.

3. **Pilot Testing:** Conducting pilot testing of the PRO measure in a sample representative of the target population can help identify any issues related to validity and reliability before full-scale implementation. This testing phase can provide insights into the clarity of the items, the appropriateness of the response options, and the overall feasibility of the measure.

Cultural Adaptation And Translation

1. **Recognizing Cultural Variability:** Health beliefs, practices, and the interpretation of symptoms can vary widely across cultures. Therefore, it is essential to adapt PRO measures for cultural relevance. Cultural adaptation ensures that the items resonate with the

target population's values, beliefs, and experiences.

2. **Translation Process:** When adapting PRO measures for non-English speaking populations, a thorough translation process is necessary. This process typically involves:
   - **Forward Translation:** A bilingual translator translates the original PRO measure into the target language, ensuring that the meaning is preserved.
   - **Back Translation:** A second bilingual translator independently translates the new version back into the original language. This step helps identify discrepancies or loss of meaning during the initial translation.
   - **Cognitive Debriefing:** Engaging members of the target population to review the translated measure provides insights into whether the items are understood as intended and culturally appropriate.

3. **Maintaining Psychometric Properties:** After translation and adaptation, it is crucial to assess the psychometric properties of the newly adapted PRO measure. This evaluation ensures that the validity and reliability of the instrument are maintained across different cultural contexts.

4. **Documentation and Transparency:** Throughout the adaptation and translation process, maintaining detailed documentation of decisions made, translation methodologies employed, and testing outcomes is vital. This transparency fosters trust and ensures that the PRO measures can be effectively utilized in diverse patient populations.

Integrating Pros Into Trial Design

Integrating Patient-Reported Outcomes (PROs) into clinical trial design is essential for capturing the patient experience and ensuring that trial results reflect the realities of living with a particular condition or undergoing a specific treatment.

Frequency and Timing of PRO Assessments

1. **Determining Optimal Assessment Points:** The timing of PRO assessments is crucial for capturing relevant data throughout the trial. Researchers should consider assessing PROs at various points, including:
    - **Baseline Assessments:** To establish a reference point, PROs should be collected before the initiation of treatment. This helps in understanding the patient's status prior to intervention.
    - **During Treatment:** Regular assessments during the treatment phase can help capture fluctuations in symptoms, side effects, and overall quality of life. The frequency of these assessments should align with the expected timeline of treatment effects or adverse events.
    - **Post-Treatment Follow-Up:** Assessing PROs after treatment completion can provide insights into long-term effects and recovery, helping to evaluate the sustainability of treatment benefits.
2. **Considering Patient Burden:** While frequent PRO assessments can enhance data richness, researchers must balance this with the burden placed on patients. Overly frequent assessments may lead to participant fatigue and affect compliance. Thus, researchers

should aim for a schedule that minimizes burden while capturing essential data points.
3. **Using Symptom and Treatment Milestones:** Timing assessments around key milestones, such as changes in treatment regimens, significant clinical events, or transitions in care, can provide valuable context for interpreting PRO data. This approach allows researchers to correlate changes in patient-reported outcomes with clinical events or interventions.

Electronic Pro (Epro) Solutions

1. **Advantages of ePRO Systems:** Electronic Patient-Reported Outcome (ePRO) solutions leverage technology to collect PRO data efficiently and effectively. The advantages of ePRO systems include:
    - **Real-Time Data Collection:** ePRO systems allow for immediate data entry, which can lead to more accurate and timely reporting of patient experiences.
    - **Enhanced Patient Engagement:** Digital platforms often provide patients with user-friendly interfaces that can enhance engagement and adherence to reporting schedules.
    - **Data Integrity:** Electronic systems can minimize data entry errors, improve data quality, and streamline the collection process by automating reminders and follow-ups.
2. **Mobile Applications and Web Portals:** ePRO systems can be implemented through mobile apps or web-based portals, offering patients flexible and convenient options for reporting their outcomes. These platforms

can also incorporate multimedia resources, such as instructional videos, to help patients understand how to complete their assessments accurately.

3. **Integration with Other Health Technologies:** ePRO solutions can be integrated with other health technologies, such as electronic health records (EHRs), telemedicine platforms, and remote monitoring devices. This integration allows for a more comprehensive view of the patient experience and facilitates data sharing between patients and healthcare providers.

4. **Data Security and Privacy:** Given the sensitive nature of health data, ePRO systems must adhere to strict data security and privacy standards. Researchers should ensure that electronic platforms comply with regulations such as HIPAA (Health Insurance Portability and Accountability Act) and GDPR (General Data Protection Regulation) to protect patient information.

Analyzing And Reporting Pro Data

1. **Data Analysis Techniques:** The analysis of PRO data requires careful consideration of the methodologies used to ensure robust and meaningful results. Common analysis techniques include:
    - **Descriptive Statistics:** Providing summaries of patient-reported data, including means, medians, standard deviations, and distributions, can help characterize the sample and highlight key findings.
    - **Comparative Analyses:** Utilizing statistical tests (e.g., t-tests, ANOVA) to compare PRO data between treatment groups or time

points helps assess the significance of differences observed.
- **Multivariate Analyses:** Techniques such as regression analysis can explore the relationships between PROs and other clinical variables, identifying predictors of patient outcomes.

2. **Reporting PRO Data:** Reporting of PRO data should be clear, transparent, and aligned with best practices. Key considerations include:
   - **Clarity in Presentation:** Use tables, graphs, and charts to effectively communicate findings. Visual representations can help convey complex data in an accessible manner.
   - **Contextualization of Results:** When reporting PRO data, it is essential to provide context regarding clinical significance. Discuss how the findings relate to traditional clinical endpoints and what they mean for patient care.
   - **Patient Perspectives:** In addition to statistical findings, integrating qualitative insights or patient testimonials can enrich the narrative and provide a more comprehensive understanding of the patient experience.

3. **Engaging Stakeholders in Interpretation:** Involving patients, healthcare providers, and other stakeholders in interpreting PRO data can enhance the relevance and applicability of findings. Stakeholder engagement helps ensure that the results resonate with those directly impacted by the research and fosters a collaborative approach to disseminating findings.

CHAPTER 6: ENHANCING PATIENT SUPPORT AND RETENTION

Patient retention in clinical trials is crucial for obtaining reliable data and achieving meaningful results. Enhancing patient support is vital not only to keep participants engaged throughout the trial but also to ensure their well-being during the process.

Comprehensive Patient Support Programs

1. **Overview of Support Programs:** Comprehensive patient support programs are designed to address the diverse needs of trial participants, ensuring they feel valued and supported throughout the study. These programs can improve patient retention rates, reduce dropout rates, and enhance the quality of data collected. Key components of effective patient support programs include:
    - **Clear Communication:** Providing participants with detailed information about the trial, including what to expect at each stage, can alleviate anxiety and encourage continued participation.
    - **Personalized Support:** Tailoring support services to individual patient needs fosters a sense of connection and belonging. This personalization can enhance the overall patient experience.

2. **Developing Patient-Centric Support Programs:** Designing support programs involves engaging with patients to identify their specific needs and preferences. Organizations can implement feedback mechanisms to gather input from participants, helping to shape support services that are both relevant and effective.

Travel Assistance And Reimbursement

1. **Importance of Travel Assistance:** Travel can be a significant barrier for many patients participating in clinical trials, especially those with chronic illnesses or disabilities. Offering travel assistance helps reduce this burden, ensuring that patients can attend their appointments without added stress or financial strain.
2. **Types of Travel Support:**
    - **Reimbursement for Travel Expenses:** Providing reimbursement for transportation costs—whether through public transport, mileage reimbursement for personal vehicles, or taxi services—can make attending appointments more manageable for patients.
    - **Transportation Services:** Some trials may offer transportation services to ensure that patients reach their appointments safely and on time. This can include ride-sharing services, shuttle buses, or partnerships with local transport companies.
    - **Accommodations for Long-Distance Travel:** For patients traveling from afar, providing accommodations can facilitate participation. This may involve partnerships

with local hotels or arrangements for lodging that minimizes the financial impact on participants.

3. **Implementation of Travel Assistance Programs:**
    - **Clear Guidelines:** To effectively implement travel assistance programs, clear guidelines should be established, outlining eligibility, reimbursement processes, and the types of expenses covered.
    - **Patient Communication:** Patients should be informed about available travel assistance options at the beginning of the trial to alleviate concerns regarding transportation.

Childcare Services

1. **Addressing Childcare Needs:** For many patients, especially parents or caregivers, the inability to secure childcare can be a significant barrier to participating in clinical trials. Providing childcare services or support can enhance patient retention and improve trial accessibility.

2. **Types of Childcare Support:**
    - **On-Site Childcare:** Offering on-site childcare at trial locations allows parents to participate in appointments without worrying about their children. This service can create a more convenient and supportive environment.
    - **Childcare Subsidies:** For trials without on-site services, providing childcare subsidies can help cover the costs associated with hiring a babysitter or enrolling children in daycare during appointments.

- **Partnerships with Local Childcare Providers:** Establishing partnerships with local childcare facilities can provide trial participants with resources and options that cater to their needs.

3. **Promoting Childcare Services:**
   - **Awareness Campaigns:** Informing participants about available childcare services should be part of the initial trial recruitment process. Clear communication about these services can encourage participation among parents.
   - **Feedback and Adaptation:** Gathering feedback from parents regarding childcare services can help refine offerings and ensure they effectively address patient needs.

Psychosocial Support

1. **Recognizing Psychosocial Needs:** Clinical trials can be emotionally and psychologically taxing for participants, especially those dealing with serious health conditions. Providing psychosocial support is crucial for maintaining participant well-being and encouraging ongoing engagement.

2. **Types of Psychosocial Support Services:**
   - **Counseling Services:** Access to counseling or therapy can help patients cope with anxiety, stress, or depression that may arise during their trial experience. Offering mental health resources as part of the patient support program can enhance overall patient satisfaction.
   - **Support Groups:** Creating peer support

groups where patients can share their experiences and connect with others facing similar challenges can foster a sense of community and provide emotional relief.
- **Educational Resources:** Providing educational materials about coping strategies, stress management, and the emotional aspects of participating in clinical trials can empower patients and help them navigate their experiences more effectively.

3. **Implementation Strategies:**
   - **Training Staff:** Ensuring that trial staff are trained to recognize and respond to psychosocial needs can create a more supportive environment for participants.
   - **Referral Networks:** Establishing referral networks with mental health professionals or organizations specializing in patient support can broaden the range of services available to participants.

Personalized Patient Engagement Strategies

In the evolving landscape of clinical trials, personalized patient engagement strategies are becoming increasingly vital. These strategies aim to cater to individual preferences and diverse needs, enhancing the overall patient experience and improving retention rates.

By recognizing that each patient is unique, researchers and trial coordinators can foster stronger connections and ensure that participants feel valued and understood throughout the trial process.

Tailoring Communication To Individual Preferences

1. **Understanding Patient Preferences:** Effective patient engagement begins with understanding the individual preferences of participants. This involves actively listening to patients and assessing their communication styles, preferred channels, and information needs. Key strategies for tailoring communication include:
    - **Surveys and Questionnaires:** Conducting pre-trial surveys can help gather information about patients' preferred communication methods (e.g., phone calls, emails, text messages) and frequency of contact.
    - **Personal Interviews:** Engaging in one-on-one conversations with patients can provide deeper insights into their preferences and establish a rapport.
2. **Customized Messaging:** Once patient preferences are understood, communications can be tailored to align with their needs:
    - **Personalized Updates:** Providing updates about trial progress, changes in schedules, or relevant information tailored to each participant can foster a sense of ownership and engagement.
    - **Adjusting Tone and Language:** Adapting the tone and complexity of communication based on the patient's background can make the information more accessible and relatable. For example, using plain language

for those less familiar with medical jargon can enhance understanding.
3. **Utilizing Technology for Personalized Engagement:** Technology can facilitate personalized communication, allowing for real-time updates and interactions:
    - **Patient Portals:** Secure online platforms can enable patients to access their trial information, receive personalized notifications, and communicate with trial staff.
    - **Mobile Applications:** Developing apps that cater to individual patient preferences can enhance engagement by offering tailored resources, reminders, and support options.

Addressing Diverse Patient Needs

1. **Cultural Competence:** Recognizing and respecting the cultural backgrounds of participants is essential for effective engagement. Cultural competence involves understanding how cultural beliefs and values influence health behaviors and perceptions. Strategies to address diverse patient needs include:
    - **Cultural Sensitivity Training:** Training trial staff to understand cultural differences can improve interactions with participants and foster a more inclusive environment.
    - **Language Services:** Providing multilingual resources, including translated documents and interpreters, can help ensure that language barriers do not impede patient understanding or participation.
2. **Accommodating Different Life Circumstances:**

Patients come from varied life circumstances that can affect their ability to engage with clinical trials. Addressing these diverse needs is crucial:

- **Flexible Scheduling:** Offering flexible appointment times can accommodate patients with job commitments, caregiving responsibilities, or transportation challenges.
- **Support Services:** Providing resources such as travel assistance, childcare, and emotional support can help address barriers that may prevent participation.

3. **Incorporating Patient Feedback:** Continuous engagement with patients through feedback mechanisms is essential for identifying and addressing diverse needs:

    - **Patient Advisory Boards:** Establishing advisory boards comprising current and former trial participants can provide valuable insights into patient preferences and experiences, guiding future engagement strategies.
    - **Regular Check-Ins:** Conducting periodic check-ins with participants throughout the trial can help identify any emerging needs or concerns, allowing for timely interventions.

4. **Empowering Patients:** Empowering patients to take an active role in their care fosters engagement and satisfaction. This can be achieved by:

    - **Shared Decision-Making:** Involving patients in discussions about their treatment options and trial-related decisions reinforces their agency and encourages commitment to the trial.

- **Educational Resources:** Providing educational materials that empower patients with knowledge about their conditions and the trial process can enhance their confidence and willingness to engage.

Retention Strategies

Ensuring high retention rates in clinical trials is vital for achieving valid and reliable results. Engaging participants throughout the trial process not only enhances their experience but also fosters a sense of commitment and loyalty.

Effective retention strategies encompass regular check-ins, appreciation efforts, the creation of patient communities, and the transparent sharing of interim results and study progress. By implementing these strategies, researchers can improve patient satisfaction and overall trial outcomes.

Regular Check-Ins And Appreciation Efforts

1. **Importance of Regular Check-Ins:** Regular check-ins are crucial for maintaining open lines of communication with trial participants. These interactions provide opportunities to address concerns, answer questions, and reinforce the significance of their participation. Key aspects of effective check-ins include:
    - **Scheduled Communication:** Establishing a routine for check-ins—whether via phone calls, text messages, or emails—helps patients feel valued and keeps them informed. A consistent schedule reassures participants that their engagement is appreciated and that the trial team is

PATIENT-CENTRIC CLINICAL TRIALS

attentive to their needs.
- **Assessing Well-Being:** During check-ins, trial coordinators can inquire about participants' well-being and any challenges they may face. This proactive approach demonstrates care and can help identify potential issues that may affect retention.

2. **Appreciation Efforts:** Recognizing and appreciating patients for their participation is fundamental to fostering loyalty and motivation:
    - **Personalized Thank-You Notes:** Sending handwritten thank-you notes or personalized messages can make patients feel special and acknowledged for their contributions.
    - **Incentives and Rewards:** Offering incentives, such as gift cards, wellness products, or discounts on health-related services, can enhance motivation and appreciation.
    - **Celebrating Milestones:** Acknowledging participants' milestones—such as completing their first visit or reaching a certain point in the study—can create a sense of accomplishment and community.

Patient Communities And Support Groups

1. **Creating Patient Communities:** Establishing patient communities fosters connections among participants, providing emotional support and shared experiences. These communities can take various forms:
    - **Online Forums and Social Media Groups:** Utilizing platforms like Facebook or

85

dedicated online forums allows patients to connect, share experiences, and offer support to one another. These digital spaces can enhance a sense of belonging and reduce feelings of isolation.
- **In-Person Support Groups:** Organizing periodic in-person meetings or events can facilitate deeper connections among participants. These gatherings provide opportunities for patients to share insights, discuss their experiences, and support one another.

2. **Benefits of Patient Communities:** Patient communities contribute to retention by:
   - **Building Trust:** Participants who feel connected to others in similar situations are more likely to stay engaged and committed to the trial.
   - **Sharing Information:** Members of patient communities can share practical tips, resources, and encouragement, enhancing the overall experience and making the trial process feel less daunting.
3. **Facilitating Peer Support:** Encouraging peer support can significantly improve participant retention:
   - **Mentorship Programs:** Pairing new participants with experienced trial veterans can provide guidance, foster a sense of reassurance, and encourage ongoing involvement.

Sharing Interim Results And Study Progress

1. **The Importance of Transparency:** Regularly sharing

interim results and updates about the study's progress fosters trust and transparency between trial sponsors and participants. This practice reinforces the value of their participation and enhances engagement.

- **Feedback on Participant Impact:** Sharing how their involvement is contributing to the research can motivate participants to remain committed to the trial. For example, if preliminary findings suggest a positive trend, communicating this can instill a sense of purpose among participants.

2. **Methods for Sharing Information:**
    - **Newsletters and Updates:** Regular newsletters that provide updates on study milestones, findings, and upcoming activities can keep participants informed and engaged.
    - **Webinars and Q&A Sessions:** Hosting informational webinars where researchers share updates and answer questions can create an interactive forum for participants. This approach allows participants to engage directly with the research team and understand the significance of their contributions.

3. **Celebrating Progress:** Recognizing progress not only keeps participants informed but also motivates continued involvement:
    - **Milestone Announcements:** Celebrating significant milestones in the trial, such as reaching enrollment goals or completing specific phases, can create a sense of community and shared achievement.

ESSAM ABDELHAKIM

CHAPTER 7: MEASURING AND IMPROVING PATIENT EXPERIENCE

Incorporating patient experience into clinical trials is essential for ensuring that research meets the needs of participants and yields valid results. By measuring and improving patient experience, researchers can enhance engagement, satisfaction, and retention, leading to more successful trials.

Patient Experience Metrics

1. **Importance of Measuring Patient Experience:** Measuring patient experience is critical for identifying areas for improvement, enhancing engagement, and ensuring that trials align with patient needs and preferences. By systematically collecting and analyzing data related to patient experiences, researchers can gain insights into the effectiveness of their engagement strategies and identify potential barriers to participation.

2. **Types of Patient Experience Metrics:** Patient experience metrics can be categorized into quantitative and qualitative measures. Quantitative metrics provide numerical data that can be analyzed statistically, while qualitative metrics offer insights into participants' perceptions and feelings. This combination of metrics can give a well-rounded view of the patient experience.

Satisfaction Surveys And Feedback Tools

1. **Designing Effective Satisfaction Surveys:** Satisfaction surveys are a primary tool for collecting patient feedback about their trial experiences. To be effective, surveys should be:
    - **Clear and Concise:** Questions should be straightforward, avoiding medical jargon to ensure that participants understand them.
    - **Relevant:** Tailoring questions to specific aspects of the trial—such as recruitment, communication, and overall experience—can yield actionable insights.
    - **Easy to Access:** Surveys should be easily accessible through various channels, such as email, patient portals, or mobile applications, to encourage participation.
2. **Key Areas of Focus:** Surveys should address several key areas to comprehensively assess patient experience:
    - **Communication:** How effectively was information communicated to participants? Were they satisfied with the frequency and clarity of updates?
    - **Support Services:** Did patients feel adequately supported throughout the trial? Were their needs addressed promptly and effectively?
    - **Overall Satisfaction:** How satisfied were participants with their overall trial experience, and would they recommend the trial to others?
3. **Feedback Tools:** In addition to traditional surveys,

researchers can leverage various feedback tools to gather real-time insights:

- **Mobile Apps:** Apps designed for clinical trial participants can include built-in feedback mechanisms, allowing patients to share their thoughts conveniently.
- **Digital Comment Boxes:** Implementing digital comment boxes on patient portals or websites can encourage ongoing feedback and suggestions.

Net Promoter Score (Nps) For Clinical Trials

1. **Understanding NPS:** The Net Promoter Score (NPS) is a widely used metric that measures patient loyalty and satisfaction by asking participants a simple question: "On a scale of 0 to 10, how likely are you to recommend this trial to a friend or colleague?" Based on their responses, participants are categorized into three groups:
   - **Promoters (9-10):** Enthusiastic participants who are likely to recommend the trial.
   - **Passives (7-8):** Satisfied participants but not enthusiastic enough to promote.
   - **Detractors (0-6):** Unhappy participants who may share negative experiences.
2. **Calculating NPS:** To calculate NPS, subtract the percentage of detractors from the percentage of promoters:

$$NPS = \% \text{Promoters} - \% \text{Detractors}$$

The resulting score can range from -100 to +100, providing a clear snapshot of overall patient loyalty and satisfaction.

3. **Using NPS to Drive Improvements:** Analyzing NPS data can highlight areas for improvement:
   - **Identifying Trends:** Tracking NPS over time can reveal trends in patient experience, helping researchers understand the impact of specific interventions or changes.
   - **Targeting Feedback:** Encouraging participants to provide qualitative feedback alongside their NPS rating can help pinpoint specific issues affecting satisfaction and loyalty.

Qualitative Assessment Methods

1. **Importance of Qualitative Assessment:** While quantitative metrics provide valuable data, qualitative assessment methods offer deeper insights into participants' experiences, emotions, and perceptions. Understanding the "why" behind patient satisfaction is essential for driving meaningful improvements.
2. **Methods for Qualitative Assessment:** Several qualitative assessment methods can be employed to gather rich, detailed feedback:
   - **Interviews:** Conducting one-on-one interviews with participants can uncover valuable insights into their experiences, motivations, and challenges. Interviews can be structured or semi-structured to allow for open-ended responses.
   - **Focus Groups:** Organizing focus group discussions can facilitate dynamic conversations among participants, revealing shared experiences and concerns. This collaborative environment encourages

participants to express their thoughts openly.
- **Open-Ended Survey Questions:** Including open-ended questions in satisfaction surveys can provide opportunities for participants to elaborate on their experiences and suggest improvements.

3. **Analyzing Qualitative Data:** To effectively analyze qualitative data:
   - **Thematic Analysis:** Researchers can identify common themes or patterns in participant responses, highlighting key areas for improvement and opportunities for enhancement.
   - **Coding:** Assigning codes to specific feedback can facilitate the organization of qualitative data, making it easier to analyze trends and sentiments.

Continuous Improvement Processes

Continuous improvement processes are essential for optimizing patient experience in clinical trials. By systematically analyzing patient feedback, implementing changes based on that input, and benchmarking against best practices, clinical researchers can create a more patient-centric environment.

Analyzing Patient Feedback

1. **Collecting Feedback:** Collecting feedback from

patients is the first step toward continuous improvement. Utilizing multiple channels, such as surveys, interviews, focus groups, and real-time feedback tools, can provide a comprehensive view of patient experiences. Researchers should ensure that feedback mechanisms are easily accessible and encourage honest and constructive responses.

2. **Data Aggregation:** Once feedback is collected, the next step is aggregating and organizing the data. Researchers can categorize feedback based on themes, such as communication, support services, and trial logistics. Using software tools for data analysis can facilitate the aggregation of qualitative and quantitative data, allowing researchers to see patterns and trends more clearly.

3. **Quantitative Analysis:** Quantitative data, such as satisfaction scores and NPS, can be statistically analyzed to identify areas of strength and weakness in the trial process. This analysis can help researchers determine which aspects of the trial are positively influencing patient experience and which need improvement.

4. **Qualitative Analysis:** Qualitative feedback, gathered through open-ended survey questions, interviews, or focus groups, provides rich insights into patients' emotions, motivations, and experiences. Thematic analysis can help identify recurring themes in the feedback, enabling researchers to understand the underlying issues that may not be evident from quantitative data alone.

5. **Identifying Actionable Insights:** The ultimate goal of analyzing patient feedback is to derive actionable insights that can drive improvements. Researchers should focus on specific, tangible suggestions from patients and prioritize them based on feasibility and

potential impact.

Implementing Changes Based On Patient Input

1. **Creating an Action Plan:** After analyzing patient feedback, researchers should develop a clear action plan outlining the changes to be implemented. This plan should prioritize changes based on their potential to enhance patient experience and improve trial outcomes. Involving cross-functional teams in this process can ensure that diverse perspectives are considered.

2. **Engaging Stakeholders:** Engaging key stakeholders—such as clinical trial staff, investigators, and sponsors—is crucial for successful implementation. Sharing insights from patient feedback can help build a collective understanding of the importance of patient-centric practices and motivate stakeholders to support proposed changes.

3. **Pilot Testing Changes:** Before implementing widespread changes, researchers may consider pilot testing new strategies in a smaller subset of the trial population. This allows for real-world evaluation of the changes and provides an opportunity to gather additional feedback before rolling them out more broadly.

4. **Monitoring Implementation:** Once changes are implemented, continuous monitoring is essential to assess their effectiveness. Researchers should track metrics related to patient satisfaction and experience to determine if the changes are having the desired impact. This ongoing assessment will inform any necessary adjustments to the implemented strategies.

5. **Iterative Improvement:** Continuous improvement is

an iterative process. Researchers should be prepared to refine and adjust strategies based on ongoing feedback and performance metrics. By adopting a mindset of adaptability, clinical trials can remain responsive to patient needs.

Benchmarking And Best Practices

1. **Understanding Benchmarking:** Benchmarking involves comparing trial performance and patient experience metrics against industry standards or best practices from other successful trials. This process allows researchers to identify areas for improvement and set realistic goals for enhancing patient engagement and satisfaction.

2. **Identifying Best Practices:** Researchers can identify best practices by reviewing literature, attending industry conferences, and networking with other clinical trial professionals. These best practices may include effective communication strategies, innovative engagement techniques, and successful patient support initiatives.

3. **Setting Performance Indicators:** Establishing clear performance indicators based on benchmarking data can help researchers set targets for patient experience improvements. These indicators should be specific, measurable, achievable, relevant, and time-bound (SMART), providing a framework for evaluating progress.

4. **Collaborating with Peers:** Collaboration with peers in the clinical research community can enhance benchmarking efforts. Sharing experiences, challenges, and successes can lead to mutual learning and inspire innovative approaches to patient engagement and satisfaction.

5. **Continuous Learning and Adaptation:** The landscape of clinical research is constantly evolving. Researchers must remain open to new ideas and techniques for enhancing patient experience. By regularly reviewing benchmarking data and adapting strategies based on emerging trends and insights, clinical trials can remain at the forefront of patient-centric research.

CHAPTER 8: ETHICAL CONSIDERATIONS IN PATIENT-CENTRIC TRIALS

The shift toward patient-centric clinical trials brings numerous ethical considerations to the forefront. While prioritizing patient preferences and experiences is crucial for improving engagement and retention, it is equally important to uphold scientific integrity.

Balancing Scientific Integrity And Patient Preferences

1. **Defining Scientific Integrity:** Scientific integrity refers to the adherence to ethical and professional standards in conducting research. This includes ensuring that studies are designed, executed, and reported in a manner that is honest, transparent, and reproducible. In the context of patient-centric trials, maintaining scientific integrity means that while patient preferences are considered, they do not compromise the validity or reliability of the research.

2. **Understanding Patient Preferences:** Patient preferences encompass the values, needs, and expectations that individuals bring to clinical trials. These can influence decisions related to trial participation, adherence to protocols, and the overall trial experience. Recognizing and respecting these preferences is vital for patient engagement, yet it can

present challenges when they conflict with established scientific protocols.

3. **Navigating Conflicts:** One of the primary ethical challenges in patient-centric trials is navigating conflicts between scientific integrity and patient preferences. For example, patients may express a desire for less invasive procedures or alternative treatments that deviate from the study protocol. Researchers must strike a balance by considering patient input while ensuring that the study design remains scientifically sound.

4. **Informed Consent and Autonomy:** Informed consent is a cornerstone of ethical research, emphasizing the importance of patient autonomy. In patient-centric trials, researchers should ensure that consent processes are transparent and allow patients to understand the implications of their preferences on trial outcomes. This may involve providing clear explanations of how their preferences will be integrated into the trial design and what potential trade-offs may exist.

5. **Collaborative Decision-Making:** Emphasizing collaborative decision-making between researchers and patients can help reconcile conflicts between scientific integrity and patient preferences. By involving patients in discussions about trial design, including their values and expectations, researchers can create a more patient-centric approach that respects both individual preferences and the scientific objectives of the study.

Maintaining Equipoise

1. **Understanding Equipoise:** Equipoise refers to the ethical condition in which there is genuine

uncertainty within the expert medical community regarding the comparative therapeutic merits of each arm in a clinical trial. In patient-centric trials, maintaining equipoise is essential to ensure that patients are not placed in undue risk or given less favorable treatment options without justification.

2. **Ethical Implications of Equipoise:** Maintaining equipoise is not only crucial for scientific rigor but also for ethical accountability. If equipoise is not present, it may compromise the ethical foundation of the trial, potentially leading to ethical violations and undermining the credibility of the research. Patient-centric trials must ensure that both patients and researchers have confidence in the legitimacy of the study design.

3. **Assessing Equipoise Throughout the Trial:** Researchers must continually assess equipoise throughout the trial, particularly as new data emerges. If interim analyses suggest a clear benefit for one treatment arm, it may necessitate reevaluating the study design to ensure that patients are not exposed to ineffective or inferior treatments. Transparency about these assessments and adjustments is key to maintaining trust among patients and stakeholders.

4. **Incorporating Patient Perspectives in Equipoise:** Patient preferences can influence the perception of equipoise. For instance, if a significant number of patients express a strong preference for one treatment over another, researchers must consider how this affects the perception of balance in the trial. Engaging patients in discussions about treatment options can help clarify their perspectives while ensuring that the principles of equipoise are upheld.

Addressing Placebo Concerns

1. **Understanding Placebo Use:** Placebos are commonly used in clinical trials to determine the efficacy of new treatments by comparing them to an inert substance. While they serve an essential role in scientific research, the use of placebos raises ethical concerns, particularly in patient-centric trials where individual patient needs and preferences are prioritized.

2. **Ethical Implications of Placebo Use:** The use of placebos can lead to feelings of deception among patients, particularly if they are unaware that they may receive an inactive treatment. This potential for mistrust can undermine patient engagement and complicate informed consent processes. Researchers must address these ethical concerns to maintain transparency and build trust with trial participants.

3. **Informed Consent and Placebo Trials:** Informed consent for placebo-controlled trials requires clear communication about the potential for receiving a placebo. Researchers should explain the purpose of the placebo, its role in the study, and the conditions under which a patient might be assigned to this group. Ensuring that patients fully understand the implications of participating in a placebo-controlled trial is crucial for ethical accountability.

4. **Alternatives to Placebo Controls:** In some cases, researchers may consider alternatives to traditional placebo-controlled designs. For instance, active-controlled trials, where a new treatment is compared to an existing standard treatment, may provide a more ethically acceptable approach while still maintaining scientific rigor. By exploring alternative designs, researchers can minimize the ethical dilemmas

associated with placebo use.

5. **Addressing Patient Concerns:** Researchers must actively engage with patients to understand their concerns regarding placebo use. Providing opportunities for patients to voice their opinions and ask questions about the trial design can foster transparency and build trust. By addressing patient concerns and incorporating their feedback, researchers can create a more ethical framework for patient-centric trials.

Privacy And Data Protection

As clinical trials increasingly embrace patient-centric approaches and incorporate digital technologies, the importance of privacy and data protection has become a focal point. Patients participating in clinical trials must trust that their personal information will be handled with care and confidentiality.

Informed Consent In The Digital Age

1. **The Evolution of Informed Consent:** Informed consent has traditionally involved a paper-based process where patients are provided with study information, risks, and benefits before agreeing to participate. However, the digital age has transformed this process. Patients now engage with consent materials online, which necessitates a re-evaluation of how informed consent is obtained and documented. This shift emphasizes the need for clear communication about data usage, storage, and sharing in a digital context.

2. **Challenges in Digital Informed Consent:** While digital platforms enhance accessibility and streamline consent processes, they also present challenges. Patients may not fully comprehend the implications of consenting digitally, particularly regarding data privacy and the potential risks of sharing personal information online. Researchers must ensure that consent documents are not only accessible but also comprehensible, using plain language and visual aids to convey complex information effectively.

3. **Interactive Consent Tools:** Innovative digital tools, such as interactive consent forms and multimedia presentations, can enhance patient understanding and

engagement. These tools allow patients to navigate through key study information at their own pace, ask questions, and confirm their understanding before providing consent. Implementing these technologies can help facilitate informed decision-making and improve patient trust in the research process.

4. **Ongoing Consent:** Informed consent should not be a one-time event but an ongoing process, especially in the digital age. Researchers should provide continuous updates to patients regarding changes to study protocols, data usage, and any potential risks that may arise during the trial. Regular communication reinforces the notion that patients have the right to withdraw their consent at any time and helps maintain trust throughout the study.

5. **Addressing Data Ownership and Rights:** Informed consent in the digital age also involves clarifying issues related to data ownership and rights. Patients should be made aware of who owns their data, how it will be used, and their rights concerning its usage. Providing clear guidelines and obtaining explicit consent for data sharing with third parties is essential for building trust and ensuring ethical research practices.

Protecting Patient Data In Decentralized Trials

1. **Understanding Decentralized Trials:** Decentralized clinical trials (DCTs) leverage technology to conduct research outside traditional clinical settings, often involving remote patient monitoring, telemedicine, and electronic data collection. While DCTs enhance patient convenience and accessibility, they also pose unique challenges for data protection and privacy.

2. **Regulatory Frameworks:** Data protection regulations,

such as the General Data Protection Regulation (GDPR) in Europe and the Health Insurance Portability and Accountability Act (HIPAA) in the United States, provide essential frameworks for safeguarding patient data. Researchers must ensure that their practices comply with these regulations, implementing necessary safeguards to protect patient information during decentralized trials.

3. **Data Security Measures:** Protecting patient data requires robust security measures, especially in decentralized settings. Researchers should employ encryption, secure data storage, and access controls to prevent unauthorized access to sensitive information. Regular security audits and risk assessments can help identify vulnerabilities and enhance data protection strategies.

4. **Patient Education and Awareness:** Patients participating in decentralized trials should be educated about data protection practices and the steps taken to safeguard their information. Clear communication regarding how data is collected, stored, and shared can help alleviate patient concerns about privacy and build trust in the trial process.

5. **Use of Anonymization Techniques:** Anonymization and de-identification techniques are critical for protecting patient data, especially when sharing information with third parties or in post-trial analyses. Researchers should implement robust anonymization methods to ensure that individual patient identities cannot be traced back to the data, thus minimizing the risk of privacy breaches.

6. **Incident Response Plans:** Despite implementing data protection measures, researchers must be prepared for potential data breaches or security incidents. Developing incident response plans that outline

procedures for addressing data breaches, notifying affected patients, and mitigating harm is essential for maintaining accountability and transparency.

7. **Patient Empowerment and Control:** Empowering patients to control their data is a vital aspect of protecting privacy in decentralized trials. Researchers should consider providing patients with tools that allow them to manage their data preferences, such as opting in or out of specific data sharing arrangements. This approach fosters a sense of ownership over personal information and enhances patient engagement.

Inclusivity And Diversity

Inclusivity and diversity are critical components of patient-centric clinical trials, ensuring that research reflects the varied experiences and needs of all populations. Engaging underrepresented groups not only enhances the validity of study results but also helps address health disparities and improves health equity.

Strategies For Engaging Underrepresented Populations

1. **Community Outreach and Partnerships:** Establishing partnerships with community organizations and leaders can facilitate trust and rapport with underrepresented populations. Collaborating with local health departments, advocacy groups, and faith-based organizations can help researchers understand the cultural and social contexts of these communities. Community outreach programs can include health fairs, informational workshops, and presentations to educate potential participants about the trial and its benefits.

2. **Culturally Tailored Recruitment:** Recruitment strategies must be sensitive to the cultural beliefs and practices of underrepresented populations. Tailoring messages to resonate with specific communities can increase engagement. This may involve using culturally relevant language, imagery, and examples in recruitment materials. Researchers should also consider the preferred communication channels for different communities, whether through social media, community radio, or local newsletters.

3. **Diverse Research Teams:** Building research teams that reflect the diversity of the populations being studied can enhance understanding and improve recruitment efforts. Diverse teams bring a range of perspectives and experiences, which can lead to more inclusive trial designs and improved interactions with participants. Moreover, having team members who share cultural or linguistic backgrounds with potential participants can help build trust.

4. **Addressing Barriers to Participation:** Identifying and addressing specific barriers that may prevent underrepresented populations from participating in clinical trials is crucial. These barriers can include socioeconomic factors, lack of transportation, fear of discrimination, and limited awareness of clinical trials. Providing practical solutions, such as transportation assistance, flexible scheduling, and comprehensive informational resources, can help mitigate these challenges.

5. **Empowering Patient Advocates:** Involving patient advocates from underrepresented communities can help amplify voices and concerns that may otherwise go unheard. These advocates can assist in shaping trial designs, recruitment strategies, and communication efforts, ensuring they align with the needs and preferences of the communities they represent.

6. **Educational Initiatives:** Education is vital for fostering understanding and interest in clinical trials among underrepresented populations. Researchers can develop educational materials that explain the purpose of the trial, the importance of diverse participation, and the potential benefits for individuals and communities. Workshops, webinars, and informational sessions can provide valuable knowledge about the research process and its

implications for health.

7. **Utilizing Technology:** Leveraging technology, including telehealth services and social media platforms, can facilitate engagement with underrepresented populations. Digital platforms can help reach broader audiences and provide accessible information about clinical trials. Ensuring that these platforms are user-friendly and available in multiple languages can enhance participation.

Addressing Health Disparities In Clinical Research

1. **Understanding Health Disparities:** Health disparities refer to preventable differences in health outcomes experienced by specific populations, often influenced by factors such as socioeconomic status, race, ethnicity, geography, and access to care. Clinical research must address these disparities to ensure equitable health outcomes and inform interventions tailored to the needs of diverse populations.

2. **Inclusive Study Designs:** Clinical trial designs should prioritize inclusivity by actively seeking participants from diverse backgrounds. Researchers should consider stratifying study samples to ensure representation of underrepresented populations. This approach not only enhances the generalizability of findings but also allows for the identification of potential differences in treatment responses among diverse groups.

3. **Monitoring and Reporting Demographics:** Collecting and reporting demographic data is essential for assessing the diversity of trial participants. Researchers should track enrollment numbers by race, ethnicity, gender, age, and other relevant factors. This

data can help identify gaps in representation and inform strategies for improving inclusivity in future studies.

4. **Engaging with Health Disparity Research:** Researchers should actively engage with existing literature on health disparities to understand the underlying causes and implications for clinical research. Collaborating with experts in health equity can provide valuable insights and guidance for designing studies that address disparities effectively.

5. **Creating Community Benefits:** Ensuring that clinical research provides tangible benefits to underrepresented populations can foster goodwill and encourage participation. This may involve offering health screenings, educational resources, or community health initiatives as part of the research process. Demonstrating a commitment to community well-being can help build trust and enhance participation rates.

6. **Advocacy for Policy Change:** Advocacy for policy changes that promote health equity is essential for addressing systemic barriers faced by underrepresented populations. Researchers can work alongside community organizations to advocate for policies that improve access to care, address social determinants of health, and increase funding for research focused on health disparities.

7. **Continuous Evaluation and Adaptation:** Ongoing evaluation of recruitment and retention efforts is crucial for understanding the effectiveness of strategies aimed at engaging underrepresented populations. Researchers should be open to feedback and willing to adapt their approaches based on what they learn from participants and community partners. Continuous improvement ensures that clinical trials

remain responsive to the needs of diverse populations.

CHAPTER 9: THE FUTURE OF PATIENT-CENTRIC CLINICAL TRIALS

As clinical research evolves, the shift towards patient-centric approaches is becoming increasingly evident. Emerging technologies are at the forefront of this transformation, providing innovative solutions to enhance patient engagement, streamline trial processes, and improve overall participant experiences.

Emerging Technologies

1. **Artificial Intelligence and Machine Learning in Patient Engagement:** AI and ML are revolutionizing how researchers interact with patients and gather insights about their needs and preferences. These technologies can analyze vast amounts of data to identify patterns and predict patient behaviors, enabling more effective engagement strategies. Here are some key applications:
    - **Personalized Communication:** AI can tailor communication to individual patients based on their preferences, medical history, and engagement patterns. For instance, chatbots can provide personalized responses to patient inquiries, making it easier for them to access information and support. This personalization fosters stronger relationships between patients and trial sponsors, leading to increased trust and

participation.
- **Predictive Analytics for Recruitment:** Machine learning algorithms can analyze historical data from previous trials to identify potential barriers to recruitment and retention. By understanding factors that influence patient participation, researchers can develop targeted strategies to engage underrepresented populations and enhance overall enrollment rates.
- **Real-time Patient Feedback:** AI-powered platforms can facilitate real-time feedback from patients, allowing researchers to monitor satisfaction levels and address concerns promptly. This continuous feedback loop enables trial sponsors to make data-driven adjustments to study protocols and improve the patient experience.

2. **Virtual and Augmented Reality Applications:** VR and AR technologies offer immersive experiences that can enhance patient education, improve consent processes, and provide virtual trial participation options. Here's how these technologies can be utilized in clinical trials:
    - **Enhanced Patient Education:** VR can simulate the clinical trial experience, allowing patients to visualize procedures, potential side effects, and the overall trial process. By providing an engaging and interactive way to learn about the trial, patients are better equipped to make informed decisions about participation. AR applications can overlay information onto real-world environments, helping patients understand the implications of their

participation more clearly.
- **Virtual Site Visits:** VR technology can facilitate virtual site visits for patients who may have difficulty traveling to trial locations. Patients can explore trial sites, meet research teams, and ask questions in a virtual environment, reducing barriers to participation. This approach not only saves time and resources but also enhances accessibility for patients in remote or underserved areas.
- **Gamification of Patient Engagement:** Incorporating game-like elements into patient engagement strategies can increase motivation and retention. For example, AR applications can offer interactive challenges or rewards for completing tasks related to the trial. Gamification can also help simplify complex concepts, making it easier for patients to understand their roles and responsibilities within the study.

Future Implications

The integration of AI, ML, VR, and AR into clinical trials presents numerous opportunities for enhancing patient-centric approaches. However, it also raises important considerations that must be addressed to ensure ethical and effective implementation:

1. **Data Privacy and Security:** As technology collects and analyzes patient data, ensuring robust privacy and security measures is paramount. Patients must have confidence that their personal information is protected, and researchers must comply with regulatory requirements regarding data handling.

2. **Equity in Technology Access:** While technology can enhance patient engagement, it is essential to ensure that all patients have access to the necessary tools and resources. Disparities in technology access may limit participation among certain populations, potentially exacerbating existing health inequities.

3. **Training and Support for Research Teams:** As new technologies are introduced, research teams must receive adequate training to leverage these tools effectively. Ongoing education and support will be crucial for maximizing the benefits of AI, ML, VR, and AR in clinical trials.

4. **Patient-Centric Technology Design:** Technology solutions must prioritize user-friendliness and accessibility. Engaging patients in the design process can help ensure that the tools developed meet their needs and preferences, ultimately improving adoption and satisfaction.

5. **Regulatory Considerations:** Regulatory bodies must adapt to the rapid advancement of technology in clinical trials. Developing guidelines that address the use of AI, ML, VR, and AR while ensuring patient safety and ethical considerations will be critical in shaping the future landscape of clinical research.

Evolving Regulatory Landscape

As the clinical research environment shifts toward patient-centric approaches, regulatory bodies worldwide are adapting to support these changes. The evolving regulatory landscape is characterized by patient-focused drug development initiatives and efforts to harmonize global standards for patient-centricity. This chapter explores the significance of these regulatory developments and their implications for clinical trials.

Patient-Focused Drug Development Initiatives

1. **Definition and Objectives:** Patient-focused drug development (PFDD) is a regulatory initiative aimed at incorporating the perspectives and experiences of patients into the drug development process. The goal is to ensure that clinical trials address the needs and priorities of patients, ultimately leading to treatments that are more effective and relevant.
2. **Key Regulatory Bodies and Guidelines:**
    - **U.S. Food and Drug Administration (FDA):** The FDA has been at the forefront of promoting PFDD. In 2012, the FDA initiated the **Patient-Focused Drug Development (PFDD) Program**, which seeks to systematically collect patient input on their experiences with diseases and treatments. This program encourages the incorporation of patient-reported outcomes and preferences into clinical trial design and regulatory submissions.
    - **European Medicines Agency (EMA):** Similarly, the EMA emphasizes the importance of patient involvement in the development of medicines. Their **Guideline on the Role of Patients in the Development of Medicines** outlines expectations for involving patients in various stages of the drug development process, from concept to post-marketing.
3. **Benefits of PFDD:**
    - **Improved Trial Design:** By incorporating patient insights, researchers can design

trials that reflect the real-world experiences and expectations of patients, leading to higher recruitment and retention rates.
- **Enhanced Relevance of Outcomes:** Understanding what matters most to patients allows for the identification of meaningful endpoints that truly reflect the benefits and risks of a treatment. This can help ensure that regulatory submissions align more closely with patient needs.
- **Increased Trust and Engagement:** Engaging patients in the drug development process fosters trust and transparency, which can enhance patient participation and cooperation throughout the trial.

Harmonizing Global Standards For Patient-Centricity

1. **Need for Global Standards:** As clinical trials increasingly involve multinational collaborations, the need for harmonized global standards for patient-centricity has become evident. Different regulatory frameworks and expectations can create challenges for sponsors conducting trials across borders, leading to inconsistencies in patient engagement and data collection.
2. **International Efforts and Collaborations:**
   - **International Council for Harmonisation of Technical Requirements for Pharmaceuticals for Human Use (ICH):** The ICH has been working to establish harmonized guidelines for the pharmaceutical industry, focusing on

patient involvement and data integrity. Initiatives such as **ICH E8 (R1)** provide recommendations for clinical trial design, including the importance of considering patient perspectives.
- **Global Coalition for Regulatory Science Research (GCRSR):** This coalition aims to facilitate global collaboration among regulatory agencies, researchers, and industry stakeholders to advance regulatory science. By sharing best practices and establishing common frameworks, the coalition seeks to enhance the incorporation of patient-centric approaches in clinical trials.

3. **Key Elements of Harmonized Standards:**
    - **Patient Engagement Guidelines:** Developing standardized guidelines for patient engagement throughout the trial process can help ensure that patient voices are consistently integrated into research.
    - **Standardized Patient-Reported Outcomes:** Harmonizing the instruments used to capture patient-reported outcomes across different regions can enhance comparability and facilitate data pooling for global studies.
    - **Cultural Adaptation of Standards:** Recognizing and addressing cultural differences in patient expectations and healthcare systems is essential for developing globally applicable patient-centric standards.

4. **Challenges and Opportunities:**
    - **Balancing Local Needs with Global**

Standards: While harmonization is beneficial, it is crucial to balance the need for global standards with the recognition of local patient populations and their unique needs. Customizing patient engagement strategies to align with cultural and regional contexts can enhance their effectiveness.

- **Adapting to Technological Advancements:** The rapid evolution of technology in clinical trials presents both challenges and opportunities for regulatory harmonization. Regulatory bodies must adapt their frameworks to accommodate emerging technologies while ensuring patient safety and data integrity.

Preparing For The Next Generation Of Clinical Trials

As the landscape of clinical research evolves towards greater patient-centricity, organizations must prepare for the next generation of clinical trials. This preparation involves building patient-centric research organizations and enhancing training and development for staff to effectively implement patient-focused approaches.

Building Patient-Centric Research Organizations

1. **Defining a Patient-Centric Culture:**
    - **Leadership Commitment:** The transformation towards patient-centricity begins at the top. Organizational leadership must actively promote and embody the principles of patient engagement and collaboration. This commitment can be communicated through mission statements, policies, and strategic plans that prioritize patient perspectives.
    - **Inclusive Decision-Making:** Engaging patients in decision-making processes not only enhances trial design but also fosters a culture of respect and collaboration. Involving patients and their advocates in research discussions can lead to more relevant trial outcomes and greater buy-in from the patient community.
2. **Establishing Patient Engagement Frameworks:**
    - **Developing Standard Operating Procedures (SOPs):** Organizations should create SOPs

that outline best practices for patient engagement throughout the clinical trial lifecycle. These guidelines should address aspects such as patient recruitment, communication strategies, and feedback mechanisms to ensure consistent application across all trials.
- **Patient Advisory Boards:** Forming patient advisory boards can provide invaluable insights during trial design and implementation. These boards can be composed of patients, caregivers, and advocacy group representatives who contribute their perspectives on study objectives, recruitment strategies, and potential barriers to participation.

3. **Integrating Technology for Engagement:**
   - **Adopting Digital Platforms:** Utilizing digital tools and platforms can facilitate real-time communication and engagement with patients. These platforms can help streamline recruitment efforts, provide updates, and gather patient feedback throughout the trial process.
   - **Utilizing Data Analytics:** Organizations can leverage data analytics to identify patient needs and preferences, track engagement metrics, and optimize trial processes. This data-driven approach can inform decision-making and enhance patient experiences.

Training And Development For Patient-Centric Approaches

1. **Creating Comprehensive Training Programs:**
   - **Curriculum Development:** Training programs should encompass the principles and practices of patient-centricity, including effective communication, cultural competence, and ethical considerations. A well-rounded curriculum can equip staff with the skills needed to engage patients meaningfully and empathetically.
   - **Role-Specific Training:** Different roles within the organization may require tailored training. For instance, clinical research coordinators may need specialized training in patient recruitment strategies, while data analysts may benefit from training on interpreting patient-reported outcomes.

2. **Fostering Continuous Learning:**
   - **Workshops and Seminars:** Regular workshops and seminars can facilitate ongoing education about emerging trends in patient-centric research, regulatory updates, and innovative engagement strategies. These sessions can also serve as a platform for staff to share experiences and best practices.
   - **Mentorship Programs:** Establishing mentorship programs can provide less experienced staff with guidance from seasoned professionals who have successfully implemented patient-centric practices. This peer support can foster a culture of learning and continuous improvement.

3. **Evaluating Training Effectiveness:**

- **Feedback Mechanisms:** Organizations should implement feedback mechanisms to evaluate the effectiveness of training programs. Gathering input from staff participants can help identify areas for improvement and ensure that training is relevant and impactful.

- **Performance Metrics:** Establishing metrics to assess staff performance in patient engagement can provide insights into the effectiveness of training efforts. Metrics could include patient satisfaction scores, retention rates, and the successful implementation of patient feedback into trial design.

CONCLUSION

As we conclude this exploration of patient-centric clinical trials, it is evident that the shift towards incorporating patient perspectives is not just a trend but a transformative approach that has the potential to enhance the quality, relevance, and effectiveness of clinical research. This transformation is vital for developing treatments that genuinely meet the needs of patients, ultimately improving health outcomes and the overall trial experience.

Key Takeaways And Best Practices

1. **Emphasizing Patient Engagement:**
    - Patient engagement is at the core of patient-centric clinical trials. Involving patients in every stage of the trial process—from design to implementation—ensures that their voices are heard, valued, and integrated into research decisions. Strategies such as patient advisory boards, focus groups, and continuous feedback mechanisms can significantly enhance engagement.
2. **Designing Patient-Friendly Protocols:**
    - Simplifying trial procedures, enhancing protocol readability, and incorporating patient input into trial design are essential for making clinical trials more accessible and appealing to potential participants. By addressing common barriers to participation and tailoring protocols to meet

patient needs, organizations can improve recruitment and retention rates.

3. **Leveraging Technology:**
    - Utilizing technology, such as telemedicine platforms, mobile apps, and electronic patient-reported outcomes, can facilitate communication and engagement between researchers and patients. Technology also allows for remote monitoring and data collection, making trials more flexible and convenient for participants.

4. **Continuous Measurement and Improvement:**
    - Regularly assessing patient experiences through satisfaction surveys, qualitative assessments, and metrics like the Net Promoter Score (NPS) can provide valuable insights into the trial experience. Organizations should embrace a culture of continuous improvement, using patient feedback to refine processes and enhance support systems.

5. **Navigating Ethical Considerations:**
    - Maintaining a balance between scientific integrity and patient preferences is crucial in patient-centric trials. Organizations must prioritize ethical considerations, ensuring informed consent and protecting patient privacy, especially in decentralized trial models.

6. **Fostering Inclusivity and Diversity:**
    - Engaging underrepresented populations and addressing health disparities is essential for ensuring that clinical research reflects the diverse patient population. By employing

inclusive recruitment strategies and culturally competent practices, researchers can broaden participation and enhance the generalizability of trial results.

Call To Action For Stakeholders In The Clinical Research Ecosystem

Transforming clinical research through patient-centricity requires a collective effort from all stakeholders within the ecosystem, including researchers, regulatory bodies, healthcare providers, and patient advocates. Here are key actions stakeholders can take:

1. **Research Organizations:**
    - Commit to fostering a culture of patient-centricity by integrating patient feedback into trial design and continuously improving patient engagement strategies. Invest in training and development programs to equip staff with the necessary skills to engage with patients effectively.

2. **Regulatory Bodies:**
    - Continue to support patient-focused drug development initiatives and harmonize global standards that promote patient engagement. Provide guidance on best practices for incorporating patient perspectives into the regulatory process.

3. **Healthcare Providers:**
    - Advocate for patient involvement in clinical trials and educate patients about the benefits of participation. Collaborate with research organizations to facilitate patient access to trials and ensure that patient needs are

prioritized throughout the process.

4. **Patient Advocates:**
    - Engage with research organizations to ensure that patient perspectives are represented in trial design and execution. Work to raise awareness of the importance of patient-centric approaches within the broader healthcare community.

5. **Patients:**
    - Take an active role in participating in clinical trials and providing feedback on their experiences. Engage with research teams and advocacy groups to share insights and drive improvements in trial processes.

ABOUT THE AUTHOR

Dr Essam Abdelhakim

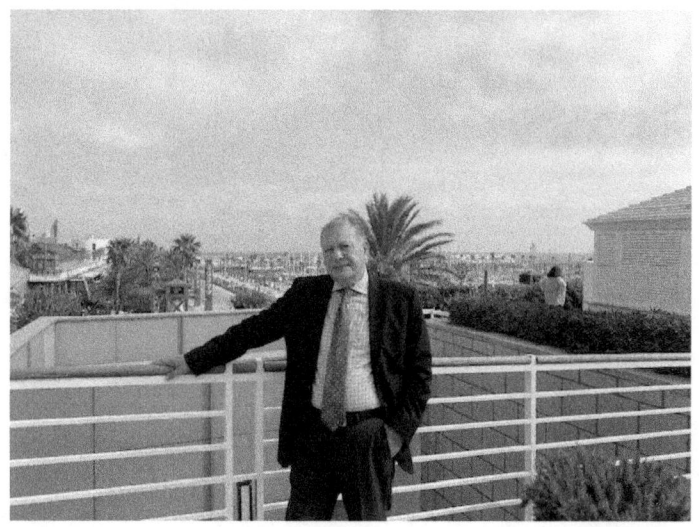

Senior Principal investigator, Expert in Clinical Research

www.ingramcontent.com/pod-product-compliance
Lightning Source LLC
Chambersburg PA
CBHW050305230526
45471CB00005B/2023